"JENNIFER KRIES' PILATES PLUS METHOD is extraordinary! Ms. Kries is an inspiration."
—*Diana F. Von Behren, Kenner, LA*

"Jennifer Kries is extremely motivating with her instruction and her routine. She understands that the whole body: mind, shell, spirit all have to be fit and conditioned. I cannot tell you what it means to feel fit, be fit, exercise regularly, eat right and feel beautiful on the inside and out. Jennifer helped me accomplish all this."
—*Deanna Dalton, Portland, OR*

"With Jennifer Kries' effective teachings, I have finally found a program that is totally right for my body and soul. It is an energizing, empowering process."
—*Colette Michaan, New York, NY*

"Jennifer's method workouts are the best! She has given me the best abs with her core exercises."
—*Ricardo Narvaez, Hockessin, DE*

"Jennifer's capacity for intuition and understanding the body is extraordinary. Her program is a lifeline to my physical well-being."
—*Max Black, New York, NY*

"Jennifer is truly connected in mind, body, and soul. She has created a way to take challenges and turn them into attainable goals."
—*Scott Featherly, personal fitness trainer, Charlevoix, MI*

"Jennifer Kries' approach to Pilates and overall mind/body fitness is unsurpassed. Her attention to detail, superb teaching style, artistry, and knowledge of anatomy makes her one of the most knowledgeable and sought after mind/body teachers. Through her work, she helps people to transform far more than just their bodies."
—*Pamela Warshay, founder/ owner of Sage Fitness for Pilates Training, New York, Master Pilates Instructor*

"JENNIFER KRIES' PILATES PLUS METHOD is what made me a true Pilates believer. The Method takes Pilates to another level. By following her program and principals you will look and feel better after the very first workout and only improve from there. Jennifer is a mind/body specialist—a visionary!"
—*Liz Neporent, author of* Fitness for Dummies *and fitness editor,* New York Times

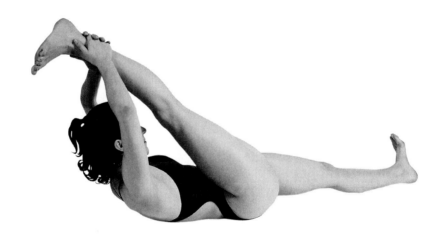

THE UNIQUE COMBINATION OF YOGA, DANCE, AND PILATES

JENNIFER KRIES'

PILATES PLUS METHOD

JENNIFER KRIES

WARNER BOOKS

An AOL Time Warner Company

Publisher's Note: Neither this exercise program nor any other exercise program
should be followed without first consulting a health care professional.
If you have any special conditions requiring attention, you should
consult your health care professional regularly regarding possible
modification of the program contained in this book.

Warner Books, Inc., 1271 Avenue of the Americas, New York, NY 10020

Visit our Web site at www.twbookmark.com.

For information on Time Warner Trade Publishing's online publishing program,
visit www.ipublish.com.

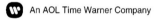 An AOL Time Warner Company

Printed in the United States of America

First Printing: January 2002

10 9 8 7 6 5 4 3 2 1

Library of Congress Cataloging-in-Publication Data

Kries, Jennifer.
[Method workout]
Jennifer Kries' Pilates plus method: a unique combination of
yoga, dance, and Pilates / Jennifer Kries.
p. cm.
Includes index.
ISBN 0-446-67734-5
1. Pilates method. 2. Exercise. 3. Yoga. 4. Physical fitness.

RA781 .K75 2002
613.7—dc21   2001035514

Book design and text composition by Jo Anne Metsch
Cover design by Brigid Pearson
Cover photograph by Ross Whitaker

To all of my students and teachers, family and friends, without whom this book would never have come to pass. Each unique interaction with you has challenged me to evolve and helped me to cultivate the ability to see more clearly, providing the fertile ground that has inspired this work. You have led me to experiment, to create, to make my contribution to the waterwheel of life, the circle that continues turning and revealing new things each time it makes its round.

ACKNOWLEDGMENTS

Diana Baroni, for opening the door, supporting my vision, and providing me with the opportunity to share my work on the printed page.

Molly Chehak, for her always-cheerful encouragement along with the design and production wizards at Warner who helped make this project such an exciting and fulfilling one.

Cal Pozo, for walking into my Mat class almost six years ago and telling me that I had to be the one to star in the first Pilates video—for making it happen. For being a pioneer in the realm of American fitness. For being a trusted friend and collaborator. Thank you!

Wendy Lipkind, for being a real friend and advisor aside from being the exceptional agent she is.

Brian Leighton for his wonderful photographs.

Patrick Quin for his room-brightening smiles and magical illustrations.

Tamah Krinsky for her impeccable taste and marvelous make-up.

Ross Whitaker and Margaret Avery for saving the day.

Emma, Henry, Olivia and Simon, Carrie and Tizzy, John and Paolo, for bringing true love, tremendous joy, and levity into my life.

My father, the gold medalist poet who was the first to teach me the importance of a good sweat.

Mama Liz, my number one fan, for her strength and admiration.

My friends, each one of them exceptional, for their love and support in all ways and for reminding me of what is truly important in life.

RJL, for his omniscience, bravery, intelligence, sensitivity, imagination, humor, spirit, and love.

My illustrious dance mentors: Joanna Wieczor, Lupe Serrano, Edward Villella, Francesca Corkle, and Mikhail Baryshnikov, for my beginnings.

The Pilates A-Team: Romana Kryzanowska, Eve Gentry, and Ron Fletcher, for passing on Joe's genius legacy.

BKS Iyengar and Alan Finger's disciples, Emily, Charles, and Jodie, for shaping my love of yoga and for helping me to learn how to breathe and how to search for inner peace.

The one and only Melvyn Hill for helping me to find it.

And finally my mother (and writing consultant), wondrous and gifted soul, for telling me many years ago that Pilates would someday come to play a significant role in my life and as a result in the lives of many others.

CONTENTS

INTRODUCTION / 1

1 · THE BIRTH OF JENNIFER KRIES' METHOD WORKOUT
3

2 · THE MAGIC TRIANGLE: Pilates, Yoga, and Dance
11

3 · THE NINE ESSENTIAL ELEMENTS
23

4 · DIPPING YOUR FOOT IN THE POOL: Pre-exercises
55

5 · THE METHOD WORKOUT
85

6 · "ON THE FLY": Sports Specifics and Time-Savers
239

7 · TAKING IT WITH YOU: THE METHOD FOR LIFE!
263

Appendix: Assessment / 271

Index / 275

Say not, "I have found the truth," but rather, "I have found a truth." Say not, "I have found the path of the soul." Say rather, "I have met the soul walking upon my path." For the soul walks upon all paths. The soul walks not upon a line, neither does it grow like a reed. The soul unfolds itself, like a lotus of countless petals.

—Kahlil Gibran,
THE PROPHET

JENNIFER KRIES'

PILATES
PLUS
METHOD

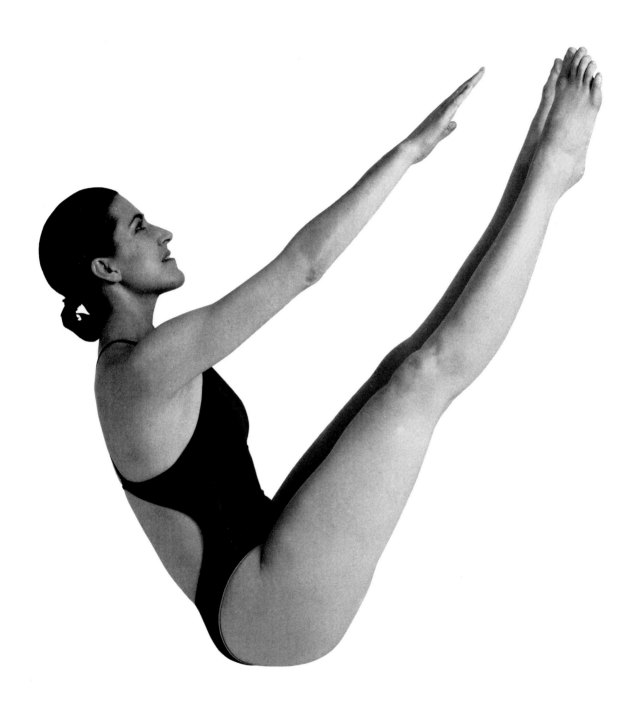

INTRODUCTION

A man travels the world over in search of what he needs,

and returns home to find it.

—George Moore

I AM AS excited about the Method Workout today as I was when I first began to weave the timeless elements that compose it. If you follow it faithfully, not only will you develop the body you always dreamed of, but you will liberate the hidden power of your mind and spirit. It will transform your life.

The Method works! It is unsurpassed in building abdominal strength, precision, and control, owing to the unique synthesis of Western athleticism and Eastern philosophy: Pilates, yoga, and dance. That is why it will continue to outlive popular trends and why it is the most sophisticated approach to physical fitness today.

The Method is not just a set of exercises that you will engage in for half-hour sessions. It is a philosophy that will improve all aspects of your life—your health, your outlook, and your state of being. This workout resource will provide you with the tools you need to realize your goals of personal achievement and excellence. I promise that this exercise program will never become a monotonous routine.

The Method relies on your brain as much as your body; it is a thoughtful and introspective approach to working out. There are no mindless repetitions, no high impact. Every movement has a purpose. Every motion has a meaning. You will focus completely on your intention, breathing, commitment, and concentration. You will become aware of your body's capabilities: strength and endurance, suppleness and flexibility. Every exercise is a technical challenge but simple to learn and fun to master. The Method builds on itself—the more you do it, the more you understand its subtleties. As in the tradition of Eastern disciplines, it becomes easier and yet more challenging at the same time. Since all of the exercises are performed against gravity, you strengthen your muscles while developing physical awareness, grace, confidence, and poise that will enhance everything you do.

Don't underestimate the power of the Method! What may at first appear to be a "workout" will turn out to be the catalyst for a dramatic change in lifestyle and profound personal transformation. The Method will transport you to a new level of awareness beyond exercise itself, to a place where your physical accomplishments are reflections of your inner victories.

The Method is designed to grow as you do. You are a unique individual with your own abilities and special needs. You will see physical and psychological results immediately, and your interest will never waiver. You will ask more of yourself and you will discover something new about yourself every day. The challenge that lies before you will be to refine and redefine your workout as you progress, to continue the quest for excellence, however elusive, to come as close as is humanly possible to the person you want to be.

You need only to open your mind and arrive at a clear understanding of why you really need and want to exercise. Then, if you are willing to entrust yourself to my care and guidance, I will be there to encourage and inspire you. I will teach you how to navigate life using art and movement as conduits for reaching higher levels of understanding and peace within yourself and in the world around you.

May this work lead you to a lifetime of fulfillment and boundless discovery.

Jennifer Kries

THE BIRTH OF JENNIFER KRIES' METHOD WORKOUT

Life isn't about finding yourself.
It's about creating yourself.
—George Bernard Shaw

M Y LOVE OF music and movement has burned inside me since I was two. According to my mother, I danced in our living room and all the neighbors used to come and watch. Even then my taste was eclectic—I loved everything from the 5th Dimension to the "Polyvetsian Dances" to Bach.

A childhood spent in countless ballet studios, including those of the Pennsylvania Ballet, finally paid off. During the summer of my thirteenth birthday, not only was I accepted to the School of American Ballet, but I stepped onto the path of my future when I signed up for "Conditioning Class" at New York City Ballet's Summer Intensive.

I remember the day I stood at the door of the studio where our classes were to be held, normally an enormous empty space. But that day, the floor was covered with foam exercise mats, lined up like soldiers in three military columns. There we were, me and fourteen other young, coltish, innocent, leotard-clad ballerinas, our hair pulled back into obedient little chignons, eyes open wide, mouths closed in expectant silence, barely breathing. Although we had all heard the expressions "Pull your tummies in" and "Derrieres under" countless times, there wasn't one among us who had any idea what those commands meant anatomically or how they would relate to what we were going to be asked to do. We would soon find out.

Then she walked in. A tall, slender, elegant woman with a twinkle in her eye and an effortless way of gliding through space. Her name was Eve Gentry. She told us that we were there to strengthen our bodies, our "centers" or our "core muscles" (abdominals), so that we could become better dancers. She told us that hard work was essential, and muscle conditioning imperative, if we wanted to prevent injury and enhance our performance in class and onstage. She told us that the "conditioning class" had been invented by her mentor and Mr. Balanchine's friend, "Joe," a man who had created a series of exercises that stretched and strengthened the body. It was a system especially intended for dancers that would help us increase our competitive edge. It would enhance our overall performance and have us jumping and turning like Baryshnikov in no time. At the mention of Baryshnikov, I was sold.

I dutifully followed Ms. Gentry's instructions. I stood at the head of my mat and crossed my arms in front of my chest. I lifted the crown of my head upward so that I appeared taller than I ever thought I could be. I used my "powerhouse," the belt of muscles extending from the buttocks up and around through the abdomen, to lower myself gracefully to the floor. I was told to lie down, lift my legs up to the ceiling, and at the same time flap my arms up and down by the sides of my body for one hundred breaths. By arm flap number twenty-five, I was in agony! I didn't think I would make it to thirty-five, let alone one hundred! I felt my abdominals for the very first time. They were burning! I could barely breathe, never mind keep my legs up and smile as Ms. Gentry commanded mercilessly, "Keep the arms pumping!" "Get the blood flowing!" "Oxygen moving!" "In and out!" "*Inhale*, two, three, four, five, and *exhale*, two, three, four, five!"

I thought I was going to die. I called my mother and told her they were torturing me. She told me to persevere. She said that the teachers knew what they were doing and that the conditioning class would soon begin to pay off.

And so I persevered. I rolled through my spine up and down on the mat, rolling like a ball, back and forth. I lifted my legs only half as often as I usually did in any of my ballet classes, and yet I felt each repetition as I never had before. I liked the precision of the movements and loved the challenge. I started to see progress. My mother was right. I was getting stronger. Within a week I could pump the arms fifty times fairly easily and balance at the end of a fancy maneuver Ms. Gentry called the open-leg rocker. One day I even rolled up into a position she called the teaser, the benchmark of the syllabus, something I thought only gymnasts or circus performers could do.

It wasn't until I returned to my regular dance schedule in the fall that I was able to appreciate the benefits I had reaped. Instead of feeling depleted after a full day of classes, I was inspired, invigorated, enlivened! My stamina had increased as well as my focus and my drive. The first day back at my three o'clock technique class, I pulled off the first triple pirouette of my career.

At the tender age of thirteen, I had been introduced to Pilates. When Eve Gentry introduced me to the "Art of Contrology" (as it was known back in the late seventies and early eighties), not only had she made me privy to an "underground exercise system," reserved for dancers and athletes, artists and performers, and society's elite, but she had bestowed on me a legacy of mind-body integration that would change my life forever.

Pilates made me feel omnipotent. I thought there was nothing I couldn't do. My range of motion and overall physical capabilities far exceeded the norm, and I pushed my body to extreme and punishing lengths. I used Pilates as a power enhancer to further exploit my body. It never occurred to me that my body would rebel. But when I seriously injured my hip while on tour in London, I was humbled and forced to reassess all that I had learned.

I discovered the Pilates Annex at the Pineapple Dance Center in London and took a class called "Rehabilitative Yoga for Dancers." I had never valued my body until I found yoga. Once I did, it profoundly changed the way I studied and lived. I learned to breathe properly—a revelation. Yogic breathing led me to a new consciousness and an awareness that my body was a vessel that deserved respect—the body is not meant to be pushed to extremes.

Upper-body strength, which I had never called upon as a ballet dancer, became mine. I had always envied people who could do push-ups. I no longer had to envy anyone. While I was becoming a more fully developed, well-rounded physical specimen, I was also becoming a more evolved and enlightened human being. For the first time I understood the value of being gentle to my body. From that point forward my body would no longer simply be a machine, distinct and separate from my mind, but would be utterly and entirely connected to it. This epiphany of mind-body integration has continued to change my life in ways I never could have anticipated. I had discovered a second exercise form that would change my life: yoga.

While I was convalescing from my hip injury, I enrolled in a teacher training program for Pilates and saw Pilates in a new light. It was not just a means of developing physical strength and power or yet another narrow approach to body conditioning. I realized that Pilates and yoga were actually ways to help rehabilitate my body.

Because I had injured myself, my body no longer responded as it always had. Even the most basic physical movements were painful, if not impossible. I was catapulted from a place where I took my body for granted: I had never thought twice about the fact that my body would perform at my will. Suddenly I was forced to learn patience, hope, courage, and determination. I learned to empathize with others' suffering, and my intuitive ability deepened. Discovering such a fascinating way to rehabilitate my body facilitated my recovery. The discovery that I was the one healing myself was integral to finding faith and rebuilding my self-confidence.

Pilates became my mantra. I knew for certain that others would benefit from it as I had. When I returned to the States, alive with triumph and new information about strengthening and healing the body, I couldn't wait to share my knowledge with others. I became a Pilates pioneer. I approached local gym facilities and introduced Pilates mat classes to the fitness public. My enthusiasm was infectious, and once people saw the phenomenal and immediate results, they were devotees.

I was once again dancing and performing regularly and began to study anatomy with renowned movement scientist Irene Dowd. Then one day my mother called—there was going to be a Pilates workshop in Philadelphia. The purpose of the workshop was to certify people in the Pilates method. There was no doubt that this would hold great meaning in my life. The instructor would be Romana Kryzanowska, a master instructor and disciple of Joseph "Joe" Pilates.

Romana was awe-inspiring. At seventy-three she could flip upside down and stand on her head! She was a phenomenon, an inspiration, a testament to what Pilates could do for the human body. She defied aging. She defied all the laws of convention. Lucky for me, she took me under her wing.

I was honored to be studying under Romana's tutelage. I apprenticed at her studio in midtown Manhattan—the notorious Drago's—where I was the beneficiary of her years of study with Joseph Pilates himself, the creator of this exercise form. She passed the torch of tradition, the legacy of Joseph Pilates, to me. I would go on to become a third-generation Pilates master teacher. Shortly thereafter, on a tour to the West Coast, I found Ron Fletcher, another exceptionally gifted Pilates disciple, and studied with him and his staff for several months. After completing more than six hundred hours on the mat and equipment, in observation and teaching, I was ready to open my first Pilates studio.

But how could I teach Pilates as I had originally learned it? How could I not share the all-encompassing philosophy of the mind-body-spirit connection I myself had begun to develop and embrace? Although I had always revered tradition and passionately embraced timeless principles, once I had woven the elements of Pilates, yoga, and dance into my own personal tapestry, my teaching would always be infused with the synthesis of the three elements and would reflect the discoveries I had made.

I began to incorporate these new elements into my teaching. People were very excited about it and my classes were always full. My students told me that they derived more from this workout—it gave them greater overall strength, flexibility, endurance, and results—than from any other. They told me they felt taller, calmer, more centered, and more secure in their bodies. They looked and felt great!

Television and radio interviews, magazine and newspaper articles, followed. There was a flood of inquiries about the work. I started to gain recognition as an innovator like Joseph Pilates himself and other exercise masters throughout history who had created movement styles and schools. Not only did my workout create a stronger, more graceful, more supple body with greater stamina and balance, but it also produced a calmer mind, a more integrated self, and an improved overall sense of well-being. The whole exercise program flowed like a carefully choreographed dance.

Jennifer Kries' Method was born.

THE MAGIC TRIANGLE: PILATES, YOGA, AND DANCE

*The real voyage of discovery consists not in seeking
new landscapes, but in having new eyes.*
—Marcel Proust

THERE IS A natural, synchronous energy that flows between the elements of what I call the magic triangle: Pilates, yoga, and dance. By incorporating these three elements, the body explores every range of motion and develops strength in every plane of movement. The power-house, the core, the breath, and the body, all moving to music, feeling release and joy! The human body is nature's miraculous design, and each element here honors that design fully.

For me, Pilates will always stand at the apex of the triangle, while yoga and dance, timeless fountains of movement and spirit, hold court in each of the other two corners. Each of these elements mirrors mutual energies and reflects shared principles while preserving its own unique identity. For example, the upper-body sculpting series and exercises are three-fourths Pilates and one-fourth yoga, a hybrid specifically geared toward enhancing upper-body strength. They are all part of the same continuum combining poetry of motion, the strength of the core (the abdominals), the rhythm of the breath—a metaphor for the body as an integrated whole.

PILATES

Pilates is a nonimpact, non–weight-bearing system of physical conditioning that focuses on body placement and increasing awareness of the body's capabilities and untapped resources. Pilates changes bodies. It makes them fitter, stronger, and more attractive. It slims the muscles and makes them longer; it develops sleekness rather than bulk. It turns the abdomen and lower back and hips into a firm, central support for a newly supple and graceful body.

Born near Düsseldorf, Germany, in 1880, Joseph Pilates (d. 1968) suffered from asthma, rickets, and rheumatic fever as a child. His determination and drive to overcome those ailments led to his study of Eastern and Western forms of exercise, including yoga and ancient Greek and Roman regimens. By the time he was fourteen, Pilates had worked so hard at bodybuilding that he was able to pose for anatomical charts and had become a diver, skier, and gymnast. When World War I broke out, he was an intern for a year in Lancaster, England, along with other German nationals. While in the camp, he taught his fellow internees the physical fitness program he had developed, and boasted that they would emerge stronger than they were before imprisonment. None of those who followed his program succumbed to the influenza epidemic that swept the nation and killed thousands. He also encountered people who were disabled as a result of wartime injuries, diseases, and incarceration, and began devising machines using the springs from old hospital beds to help in their rehabilitation. These machines were the prototypes of the equipment used in Pilates studios today.

After the war, Pilates returned to Germany to continue his work. In 1925 his teaching came to the attention of the German government. He was invited to train the New German Army but opted to try his luck in America instead. In 1926 Joseph Pilates and his wife, Clara, a nurse, brought his revolutionary method of physical and mental conditioning to the United States.

When the couple opened a studio in New York City, it caught the atten-

In 10 sessions you will feel better. In 20, you will feel better and in 30, you will have a completely new body.
—Joseph Pilates

tion of the dance community and high society alike. Pilates believed that the "attainment and maintenance of a uniformly developed body with a sound mind, fully capable of naturally and efficiently performing daily tasks with spontaneous zest and ease" should be the objective for people of all ages and fitness levels.

Pilates exercises make people more aware of their bodies. Pilates helps to improve alignment and breathing and increases efficiency of movement. The focus is on the center of the body—the "powerhouse," or the "corset muscles," also known as the integral core muscles of the torso, which include the following primary abdominal muscles:

1. the rectus abdominus and transversus abdominus
2. the internal and external obliques and pyramidalis
3. the muscles of the sides, or upper waist (teres major, infraspinatus, and serratus anterior)
4. the muscles of the back (latissimus dorsi and rhomboids) and buttocks (erector spinae, quadratus lumborum, and gluteus maximus)

Pilates has tremendous application for injury prevention because it prepares the body for balanced, efficient, and graceful movement in all spheres and ranges of motion. Pilates has addressed the needs of dancers and superathletes for decades—imagine what it can do for you!

Many athletes use it as a basis for cross-training in order to balance their own narrow training regimes. Golfers, tennis players, skiers, swimmers, and runners all benefit. Whatever your chosen sport, or even if you are simply interested in overall health and fitness, when the focus of your workout is on strengthening the power of the core (and you learn how to initiate all of your movement patterns from it), not only will you work the deeper muscles together and improve your coordination and balance, but you will reeducate yourself to focus on the present moment and the mind-body interaction (see chapter 5).

Pilates was the beginning of my introduction to the body as a "thinking machine," and the idea was revolutionary for me. Until then I had used my mind strictly to drive my body, unsympathetically directing it toward higher and higher levels of accomplishment. I never considered that I might be pushing myself too hard. Once I began to treat my body with greater care and infuse my training regime with improved balance, I accomplished a great deal more.

The Pilates exercises you will find in this book are composed of the complete, classical, original workout developed by Joseph Pilates. Pilates mat work, an ordered series of exercises that focus on the abdominal center and muscles of the torso, as well as breathing patterns for each exercise, will teach you how to direct energy to those targeted areas while relaxing the rest of your body. Because you will be doing the fewest number of repetitions with the greatest precision and control, you will

1. increase muscular definition and capacity in the legs and hips;
2. improve overall flexibility and the refinement of proper placement and postural stance;
3. develop equal strength symmetrically around the center to align the body and enhance its efficiency;
4. stretch and strengthen muscles;
5. open the joints and release tension;
6. sculpt your body, creating long, lean, beautifully toned and proportioned muscles.

Pilates works many of the deeper muscles together, improving coordination and balance. The workout is concerned with the process itself. You will learn to focus on the present moment and the movement itself rather than the outcome. This is a workout, a regime that promotes and facilitates evolution of the self more than any other.

The subtle magic of Pilates is that the work will grow as you do. You rise to higher and higher levels as your self-awareness and experience deepen. As you gain insight and as your actual physical strength increases, the work will refine and redefine itself. Exercises rely on your own individual level of strength, so they will increase in difficulty only as your body develops the ability to take on greater challenges.

My love of Pilates began long before its era of popularity and has served as a pillar of strength for me in all aspects of my professional athletic and artistic life. The body I have created and the level of personal excellence I have achieved have come, however, as the result of a special synthesis of more than just Pilates. Pilates was the foundation, an integral component, but equally important were my practice of yoga and all of my years as a professional dancer.

YOGA

> Worry means always and invariably inhibition of associations and loss of effective power. The turbulent billows of the fretful surface leave the deep parts of the ocean undisturbed, and to him who has a hold on vaster and more permanent realities the hourly vicissitudes of his personal destiny seem relatively insignificant things.
>
> *William James*

Yoga is the oldest of the physical disciplines. It is an immortal art, science, and philosophy. It is the true union of will with spirituality—the disciplining of the intellect, the emotions, the body, and the mind. Through yoga you can deeply connect to your innermost self and rise above worldly concerns and daily minutiae. You can find a place of detachment where the body and mind are one.

Yoga is about feeling centered, emotionally and spiritually grounded. It has provided me with a subtle, quiet, and introspective means of listening to my body. Once I started moving quietly and slowly through yoga, I was actually able to experience my body as an anatomical structure. I understood how and why my body moved, in a way I was not able to in Pilates or dance, both of which are performed at a faster pace.

I never realized what my body was capable of until I found yoga. Until then I had never experienced the mind and the body as an integrated whole. Yoga was the answer, the balancing element that had been missing from my regimented pursuits of Pilates and dance, both of which demanded precision and perfection. Yoga offers freedom, suppleness, and flexibility, a devotion to oneself, and greater peace of mind.

For the yoga-inspired exercises of the Method, I have drawn upon the ancient sources of hatha, Iyengar, and ashtanga. Each of these yoga techniques was developed by a different yogi, and each has its own unique characteristics that contribute to the series in the Method Workout.

In yoga you aren't expected to execute anything perfectly, to adhere to rigid, achievement-oriented strictures, or to use your body as a tool to accomplish more and more and more. The premise of yoga is kindness, compassion, and respect for the self. Yoga means patience and careful attunement to the subtle whisperings of the body. The spirit is nurtured by respecting one's body, by becoming closer to it. By establishing an environment that fosters celebration of the self, of your body exactly as it is, you actually cultivate the ability to release your preconceived notions of what your body "should" be capable of or what it "should" look like and to give up those desires. In giving yourself permission to experiment, in giving yourself over to the breath, you gain some distance from yourself, from your physical concerns, and free your mind. Inevitably, you find a space that permits you to focus on the more important aspects of your life— finding true balance and peace in your body in the present moment. The very nature of yoga is gentle and slow and steady, and through following the rhythm of the poses in your practice, your perspective is positively altered and your mind is slowly, almost imperceptibly calmed. Through yoga you can connect to your innermost self and achieve profound union of mind and body, reaping the benefits that lie in the subtle workings of the breath and the asanas (postures or poses).

Yoga begins with the breath. The breath leads the body and calms the mind. You will learn to breathe in a way that will profoundly influence every day—the way your body functions, the way your mind works.

Breathing is the way to access the meditative mind. There are three kinds of breathing:

1. alternate nostril breathing, which is meditative and reflective;
2. ujjayi, the breath of concentration; and
3. kapalabhati, the breath of fire.

Learning these techniques will teach you that the breath is a powerful healing force and that, as in the Chinese art of acupuncture, it can open or create new pathways where vital energy *chi* can flow. Where once there were restrictions, yogic breath coaxes the body into opening and releasing unavailable or locked-up energy so that equilibrium can be established. If there is restriction in the body, that means vital energy (*chi*) is blocked and participation from that particular area is diminished. The ancient Chinese art of acupuncture is remarkably effective in this aspect; through the insertion of tiny needles carefully targeted along the body's meridians (energy pathways), the body is coaxed into relinquishing its holding patterns, and balance is restored. Amazingly, through yogic breathing, you can achieve the same effects. When you are able to breathe deeply and completely, the breath itself becomes a gentle, catalytic force helping you to move into territories of your body you have never explored before. You don't have to be a world traveler, for once you truly learn how to breathe and explore your capabilities through yoga, your body's topography and geography become the most exciting new land you could discover.

Yoga asanas (postures) strengthen the upper body in a way that surpasses Pilates or weight lifting alone. Whereas Pilates focuses primarily on increasing strength in the center and on overall symmetry (proportionate strength throughout the entire body), and weight lifting builds strength through muscular isolation, yoga emphasizes integrative upper-body strength through continuous movement patterns that rely heavily on the muscles of the arms, chest, shoulders, and back. From the beginning of the asana series, in the Sun Salutation, the body is asked to support its own weight with the hands and arms and is required to push off the floor in order to move smoothly through the postures. As a result, all the muscles of the upper body develop strength, stamina, definition, and control.

I believe the yoga postures will inspire you as they have me to achieve a healthier balance between mind and body, relieve a host of physical ailments, and cope with the stresses and strains of your everyday life. The postures and techniques I have chosen will not require a lifetime of dedication and practice but are accessible to everyone, no matter your age, health, or life circumstance. With yoga you will integrate the body, mind, and spirit. You can profoundly influence the way your body functions, the quality of your everyday life, the workings of your mind.

You can find a place of detachment where the mind and body are one. Where the spirit is nurtured. Begin with the breath. It is the breath that leads the body and calms the mind. It is the breath that quiets the mind and heals the body.

DANCE

As we discussed in the yoga section, when the mind and body are in concert with one another, you will discover a lighter, more buoyant, more resilient spirit.

Nothing can better express this resilient spirit than the euphoric, almost trancelike feeling of transcending the body in dance. While Pilates and yoga may share elements in common with it, dance develops overall stamina, endurance, and determination. It is dance that creates a better-looking body; regal posture that is second nature; natural grace and poise; long, lean, elegant muscles; spatial awareness; and strength.

I own a sense of discipline that touches every aspect of my life. I have often taken it for granted, but dance has always provided me with the formula to achieve. Dance demands an almost superhuman discipline, sacrifice and commitment to the highest standard of excellence. It demands perfection. Even the most basic exercises in the classical ballet syllabus inspire exactitude; no other modality requires such precision and control. Dancers are the ultimate athletes. But don't worry, the dance elements I've used in the Method Workout will not require superhuman qualities of you. I have chosen a collection of the most basic ballet and modern dance warm-up exercises that is challenging yet accessible; the exercises will provide you with a perfectly well-rounded introduction to dance and will help you to sculpt the body of your dreams. The elements I have included in the workout will still bestow the same physical results as if you were a professional dancer yourself.

Dance, the instinctual, universally human expression, takes the body through music and movement to another, higher dimension: increased muscular stamina; heart-strengthening, body-strengthening, inconceivable motion. Paradoxically, as you invest your every ounce of effort in its potentialities, always pushing the envelope, tirelessly raising the bar one step higher, struggling to physically manifest your personal image of perfection, you are somehow, miraculously, able to lose yourself to the music. . . . You forget your body, you forget the effort, you forget yourself.

Traditional dance classes feature three segments: a warm-up; a combination, or workout; and a cool-down. The warm-up is both a study and a practice of the basic strength techniques and movement patterns that will later connect to become longer movement patterns. Beginners and seasoned dancers alike warm up with the same exercises. In fact, long after dancers leave the stage and are no longer dancing professionally, they often continue to keep their bodies in shape by attending the warm-up segments of dance class.

The dance-inspired exercises of the Method are based on a blend of classical ballet and modern dance, a typical contemporary dance warm-up. They feature simple movements that target specific muscle groups, conditioning and strengthening the body through contraction and release. An array of the most effective body-sculpting techniques, they create an integrated, mobile awareness of the muscles we use for abdominal support and proper body alignment.

I will take you through smooth, continuous, choreographed segments that will free your body and leave you feeling energized, motivated, and proud. The result will be increased physical strength and endurance, greater focus and stamina. You will cultivate a feeling of length and poise and an unrivaled sense of accomplishment. There is no other exercise modality that can boast both the sense of groundedness and the sense of weightlessness that one experiences in dance.

Pilates, yoga, and dance: the perfect combination for mind, body, and spirit. Together, with your commitment and concentration, these three components of the magic triangle create the alchemy of change that will help you to transform your life in ways you never anticipated.

THE
NINE
ESSENTIAL
ELEMENTS

The Tao of nurturing life requires that one keep oneself

as fluid and as flexible as possible. One should not stay still for too long,

nor should one exhaust oneself by trying to perform impossible tasks.

One should learn how to exercise from nature by observing

the fact that flowing water never stagnates and a busy

door with active hinges never rusts or rots.

Why? Because they exercise themselves

perpetually and are almost always moving.

—Sun Ssu-mo

I F YOU HAVE picked this book up off the shelf, you must be searching for a new way to care for and improve your body. You are looking for an exercise program you can follow faithfully, one that will change your body and deepen your experience of your own true self. The Method Workout is for you.

If you are like most people, you may benefit from personal attention and support during your quest. I will be your guide and your companion as you work your way through the pages of this book and as you evaluate what your starting point should be. If you are attentive and willing to entrust yourself to my care and guidance, mine will be the voice of reason, the voice of assessment and encouragement you hear whispering in your ear. You will feel my presence as if you were actually taking a class with me, as if we were really together. I will help you to embrace the Method Workout and teach you how to benefit from all of its elements, but it is you who will assimilate the twists and turns of each exercise you choose to add to your repertoire. You who will weave your own tapestry with your own special colors, textures, and threads.

THERE ARE NINE essential elements that form the foundation of your body's new memory and will prepare your mind and body for all that lies ahead. They are the quintessential and underlying principles of the Method, as well as the preschool for all the Method workouts. Inherent in all the elements and every exercise you will do in the Method Workout is a special combination of concentration, control, flowing motion, precision, and imagination. Concentrating over a period of time on the elements, combined with special attention to the breath, results in the growth of a powerful sense of well-being and confidence. Learning, growth, and integration—like the changes in the shape of your body—are brought about by the activity itself, without conscious stress on the goals. The essential elements lie at the heart of the heightened physical and emotional power we are striving to attain. These are the Nine Essential Elements:

1. Breathing
2. Establishing the navel-to-spine connection
3. Effortless effort
4. The principle of opposition
5. Quality versus quantity
6. Intuitive integration
7. Transitions
8. Tempo and dynamic
9. Meditation

Once you begin to understand these elements intellectually, I will teach you how to physicalize and actualize (or practice and master) each one of them until they have become second nature to you, and you yourself believe them to be an essential part of whatever you do. I promise that you will derive unparalleled physical and spiritual satisfaction from the focus and concentration required to perform them.

During my explanation of each of the Nine Elements, I will outline instructions and give you exercises to help you understand each. These exercises will help you to enhance your overall workout, which we will get to in chapter 5. If you are willing to invest the time it takes to understand

and master these fundamental and essential elements, not only will you gain great advantage when you are ready to begin the Pre-exercises in chapter 4 and the actual workouts in the following chapter, but the purity and the simplicity of the elements themselves will be their own reward. And now, let's begin!

I. BREATHING

If you never wholly give yourself up to the chair you sit in, but always keep your leg- and body-muscles half contracted for a rise; if you breathe eighteen or nineteen instead of sixteen times a minute, and never quite breathe out at that,—what mental mood can you be in but one of inner panting and expectancy, and how can the future and its worries possibly forsake your mind? On the other hand, how can they gain admission to your mind if your brow be unruffled, your respiration calm and complete, and your muscles all relaxed?

William James,
—*"The Gospel of Relaxation"*

Breathing is something we usually take for granted. Unlike Eastern civilizations, where breathing is regarded as a science, we in the West have attributed little importance to it. China has its *qi gong* (pronounced *chee gung*), and India its *pranayama.* But most of us breathe without any consciousness of the process. It is something we do from the moment we are born to the moment we die.

Learning to control the way we breathe is fundamental to the Method. The rhythm of the breath, breath and energy, breath and the emotions, and the power of the core are all inextricably linked. With a little patience and practice the lungs, the diaphragm, the abdomen, and the circulatory system welcome the rigors of deep breathing. This duet of breath and energy forms the bridge between body and mind.

What distinguishes ordinary, everyday breathing from deep abdominal breathing is the diaphragm. It is truly the workhorse of the breathing mechanism of the body. The deep abdominal breathing we focus on in the Method will stretch and strengthen this resilient, flexible muscular membrane in addition to strengthening your core abdominal muscles. Every time the lungs expand in a deep breath, they push the diaphragm downward. Each time the lungs contract in an exhalation, the diaphragm is pulled up into the chest cavity. The diaphragm really acts like another heart.

Almost every part of your body, from the muscles in your upper neck, starting at the base of your skull, and going all the way down to your lower back and sacrum, involves itself in the breathing process. Every time you inhale, the muscular structures in the neck and shoulders help to lift the rib cage in order to accommodate the lungs' expansion. The movements of the rib cage itself are dynamic; it moves not only in and out but up and down, front and back.

Have you ever realized that you can send your breath almost anywhere? When you explore where your breath can travel by using your hands (by placing your hands on your rib cage, chest, and stomach), you can feel some of the more obvious places it goes, but you haven't begun to know the parts of your body you can breathe into! You can send breath to places that are less accustomed to receiving that kind of care, such as your upper back, your lower back, the sides of your ribs, your neck. Places that suffer from restrictions can benefit tremendously from some focused breath attention. Sending fresh oxygen to injuries or tight muscles can help them loosen and become more flexible, reinvolve them in the breathing dynamic, and make your breathing more efficient.

In becoming more aware of how your body works during the breathing process, you will learn to maximize your efforts when you inhale, exhale, and retain breath, and when you acquire and practice the more involved breathing techniques that stand at the core of the Method Workout.

You know that feeling that hits you at the end of a long workday. The clock strikes five and you glance over at your gym bag and then at the invitation to a cocktail party that sits seductively on your desk.

"No contest," the devil in your head barks. "You're tired! You've worked hard all day, and a martini with a twist, no olives, sounds great!"

The angel in your head is flapping tirelessly, smiling that beneficent, benign smile. "You'll feel so much better if you just make it down to the gym and put in an hour on the treadmill! Think of how great you'll look in that new Armani dress!"

Suddenly the angel's wings are wilting and you're ready to grab the martini from the devil's hand. There's no air in your office and your eyelids are fluttering.

What's the lesson here? Sure, you've worked hard all day. But more to the point, you probably haven't taken in a full, complete breath all day. If you had, you'd be excited to put the contents of your gym bag to good use instead of strolling down devil's lane.

Most people are not even aware of the importance of breathing, that without sufficient oxygen we become fatigued and lethargic. For optimum health, breathing should be consistent, full, and rhythmic, using the diaphragm and ribs to fill and empty the lungs. The complete change of air in the lungs increases oxygen levels in the body, which produces energy. Toxins are eliminated, fresh air is brought in to replace stale, circulation improves, mental clarity and concentration increase, your general outlook improves, and a sense of equilibrium is restored—all from breathing properly!

In yoga classes it is not uncommon to hear the teacher say, "Now we will breathe to balance the right and left sides of our brain, the yin and yang of the body." What the teacher is really describing is integrating the sympathetic and the parasympathetic, the two branches of the nervous system, which, like yin and yang, are both antagonistic and complementary to one another. When the sympathetic nerves are activated in preparation for physical and mental activity, the pulse increases, adrenaline is stimulated, and respiration is heightened. When the parasympathetic branch is activated (which controls vital functions such as digestion, elimination, and metabolism), the "action" circuits shut down and the entire body is calmed. When you breathe deeply and properly, you are able to balance and mediate between these two control centers. Deep breathing calms the emotions and reestablishes a natural balance between the two, making it a highly effective and preventive therapy against the stresses and strains of our everyday lives.

There are as many different ways to breathe as there are to dance, each with its own rhythm, beat, and style. For our purposes, we are going to keep it simple and incorporate but a few. In the Method Workout, we will incorporate the following breathing techniques:

1. *Kapalabhati,* the breath of fire, the foundation for the Hundred breath and warming up
2. *Retention,* with the three locks, to increase lung capacity and strengthen the heart
3. *Ujjayi,* the smooth concentrated breath for all the yoga poses
4. *Basic inhalation and exhalation with abdominal contraction,* for all the Pilates exercises
5. *Alternate nostril breathing* for final meditation

Inhalation

The word *inhalation* was once synonymous with *inspiration,* reminding us that even in Western civilization the intimate links between breath and spirit were once acknowledged. During inhalation, in purely physical terms, the chest expands and the lungs are filled with fresh air. But in the greater sense, inhalation signals the intake of vital energy—the body's equilibrium and coherence, its activity and creativity, are all established through inhalation, the primary life-giving force.

EXERCISE 1: LEARNING TO BREATHE

Sit comfortably in your chair. With abdomen relaxed, shoulders loose, and spine erect, inhale deeply and then simply empty your lungs completely with an exhalation. Now I'm going to ask you to use your sense of touch to locate exactly where your breath goes when you breathe naturally and where it can go when you direct it.

Place your hands on your belly and feel it expand as you inhale. As you exhale, feel the abdomen relax back to its natural state. As you take your second inhalation, move your hands to your rib cage and feel the ribs expand as you inhale and how they return to their normal state when you exhale. Move your hands on to your chest, and when you inhale again, feel the rise of your chest as it expands to accommodate the new intake of air. As you exhale, feel your chest fall and return to its natural state. Before you inhale this time, try pulling your navel toward your spine (more on how to do this in the next element) and feel how you are sending the breath primarily to your chest. Can you see how different that inhalation was? How much more challenging it is to take in the same amount of air as you did when you allowed the breath to go to your belly!

IN MOST OF the Method workouts, you will be maintaining this navel-to-spine connection as you breathe. Not only will you increase your lung capacity by sending the air higher up into your chest, but you will tone and strengthen your abdominal muscles as well.

Retention

Retention is the act of holding your breath and using your body as a container for the breath, which you store temporarily in a focused way. When you inhale deeply and hold or prolong a breath, you profoundly benefit every organ, gland, and functional system in the body. Even during a brief retention, the heartbeat slows, blood pressure is reduced, and cells throughout the body begin to "breathe" by themselves. The heat and perspiration you feel after ten to fifteen minutes of deep breathing and breath retention exercises testify to this enhanced cellular respiration. Likewise in the lungs, retention enriches the blood with extra oxygen and purges it of extra carbon dioxide by prolonging the time for gas exchange.

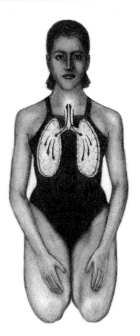

Inhalation

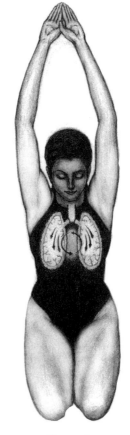

Retention

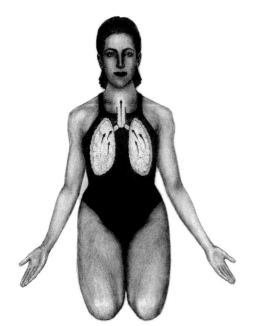

Exhalation

Breath retention increases the pressure of oxygen against the capillary walls in the tissues, enhancing gas exchange between bloodstream and cells as well.

EXERCISE 2: UNDERSTANDING RETENTION

Sitting comfortably in your chair, inhale deeply through your nose and then exhale completely. Inhale once again, allowing your abdomen to expand naturally, but inhale only to a comfortable place, not as deeply as the first time. As you inhale, sweep your arms up by your sides, up and over your head, and link your thumbs together, dropping your chin to your chest. With eyes closed, hold your breath for as long as you comfortably can. Imagine while you are doing this that new cells are being born. When you cannot hold your breath any longer, unlock your thumbs, lift your chin, and open your eyes and slowly exhale through your nose as your arms float down by the sides of your body and come to rest on your lap.

WHEN YOU WANT to safeguard important documents, jewelry, and other valuables, what do you do? Lock them up! Absolutely! And that is exactly what we are going to learn how to do with one of our body's most precious possessions: the breath.

Retention and the Three Locks

We use the "three locks" (otherwise known as "energy bath stoppers") to maximize the retention of the breath. The anal lock, the abdominal lock, and the throat lock are used separately or in combination to create a therapeutic compression of breath within the abdominal cavity. Not only does this expand the walls of the alveoli (tiny air sacs) in the lungs, thereby increasing lung capacity and stamina, but also, by virtue of creating this void or *window of perfect stillness* within, circulation is enhanced, the nervous system is calmed, and precious *chi*, or vital energy, is gathered.

The Anal Lock (Mula Bhanda)

When the diaphragm descends into the abdominal cavity with an inhalation, the anal lock (or "mula bhanda," as it is known in yoga breathing practices) raises the pelvic floor. The breath just inhaled is compressed and "locked in" or retained.

Just as the inhalation phase approaches completion, the anal lock is applied by contracting the perineum (the band of muscle in the urogenital region). The energy of that breath is sent deep into the abdominal cavity and held there. Internal pressure increases, and in combination with the other two locks (abdominal and throat), circulation increases and blood is exchanged in the internal organs and surrounding tissues.

EXERCISE 3: MULA BHANDA

Sitting comfortably, inhale, and just as you begin to hold the breath, contract the outer ring of the anal sphincter (the tough band of muscle that controls the external aperture of the anus and the perineum), thereby lifting the entire webbing of the urogenital region. Squeeze this region, without exerting too much pressure, and appreciate the subtle stimulation and lift that the contraction creates in your lower body. Retain the breath for as long as you comfortably can, and then, as you exhale, gently release the anal lock.

The Abdominal Lock

The second lock is also used to seal in the therapeutic compression, but this time it is located in the center of the abdominal cavity. When the abdominal lock (and the abdominal wall) combines with the anal lock, not only does it encourage massage of the internal organs and glands, but it creates a powerful propulsive force that pushes blood up into the chest just like a pump. The heart is temporarily relieved of its normal workload. Brief moments like these—of enhanced abdominal and urogenital contraction—save your heart a substantial amount of work. In fact, while you are maintaining your retention, you will be more sensitive and sympathetic to the beat of your heart and its natural function. You will feel your heart slow down and beat in a more deliberate way. Imagine if you were to practice this breathing technique even a few times a week how it would enhance the health and work life of your heart.

EXERCISE 4: THE ABDOMINAL LOCK

With arms long at your sides, sitting with the body tall and relaxed, inhale until you feel that your lungs are nearly full. Then apply the abdominal lock by pulling the lower part of the abdominal wall inward toward the spine (remember the tight-jeans scenario; where you have to pull your navel to your spine, away from the waistband, in order to zip the jeans?). Hold this contraction for the duration of your retention. Hold your breath for as long as you can without strain or discomfort, and as you begin to exhale, release the abdominal contraction.

The Throat Lock

The last of the three locks, the throat lock, serves many functions. When you constrict the throat area, blood is diverted and distributed to the lower extremities for a more balanced circulation. The throat lock seals the breath down inside the lungs after you have inhaled so that it doesn't rise up and cause uncomfortable pressure in the throat, nostrils, and eustachian tubes during compression. Finally, the action of dropping the chin forward slightly onto the chest creates a gentle traction for the spinal column—the entire spinal cord from the skull to the sacrum is stretched, stimulating all the muscles and nerves that run along its length.

EXERCISE 5: THE THROAT LOCK

To apply the throat lock, sitting comfortably in your chair, contract the throat muscles and clamp the glottis over the trachea (put more simply: constrict the back of the throat). Can you feel it? Release. Now let's begin:

Inhale completely while contracting the back of the throat. At the end of the inhalation, tuck your chin in slightly toward your chest and stretch the back of your neck, bending it somewhat forward without sacrificing the length in the upper spine. Your shoulders are still relaxed, the chest is expanded, and the neck is long.

Hold the breath for as long as you comfortably can, focusing on the breath and the energy circulating, locked inside you. When you are ready to exhale, when you feel that you can no longer comfortably contain the breath, raise your chin so that your eyes are focused straight ahead and let the air flow gently out through your nose or mouth by forming a whistle shape with your lips, directing the breath toward a point in front of you.

Exhalation

In simple terms, exhalation rids the body of stale air to make way for fresh air. According to B. K. S. Iyengar's *Light on Pranayama,* "exhalation is the outflow of individual energy which quiets and silences the brain. . . . In exhalation, all thoughts and emotions are emptied with the breath."

Exhalation occurs at the end of the cycle, but it may also be seen as the beginning; it makes way for the blank canvas that awaits fulfillment, the empty vessel into which inspiration and vitality are breathed.

EXERCISE 6: EXHALATION

This time, as you inhale, I would like you to imagine that you are expanding into a big red, round, happy balloon. Then, with one hand on your chest, the other on your belly, begin to exhale. Feel the air go out of the "balloon" from the top down. First the chest returns to its relaxed state and then, deflating and traveling downward, the stomach. See yourself, the big red balloon, quietly, slowly letting go of all the air that has filled you. You will be emptying the lungs in reverse order of inhalation. At the end of the exhalation, if you are able to, pull the entire abdominal wall inward in order to expel the last residues of stale air from the lower lungs, leaving an empty vessel to make way for a fresh, new intake of air—a new opportunity for expansion. This final contraction of the abdomen also compresses the inner organs and disgorges the extra blood pumped into them during inhalation.

Now, let's combine everything we've learned about breathing.

EXERCISE 7: FULL INHALATION, RETENTION WITH THE THREE LOCKS, AND EXHALATION

Sitting comfortably in your chair, inhale deeply through your nose and exhale completely. Inhale again but not as deeply as the first time you inhaled—this time inhale to a more comfortable place, allowing your abdomen to expand naturally. Picture the breath as it swirls within your expanded abdomen and imagine all the healthy rewards.

As you inhale, sweep your arms up by your sides and UP over your head, and as you do this, apply the anal lock, then the abdominal lock, and link your thumbs together.

Drop your chin to your chest as you apply the throat lock, and with eyes closed, hold your breath for as long as you comfortably can. As you do this, imagine all the cells that are being born. You are so generously oxygenating your system!

When you can no longer hold your breath, unlock your thumbs, as well as the three locks, lift your chin, open your eyes, and slowly exhale through your nose as your arms float down by the sides of your body and come to rest in your lap. WOW!!! WELL DONE!!!

Note: *NEVER hold your breath beyond what feels comfortable! If you have gasped or burst out your breath on the exhale, it means you have held the retention too long and lost control of your breath.*

The Rhythm in Your Breathing

The mind is naturally attracted to rhythm. That is why the rhythmic breathing techniques we use in the Method will add value to every exercise you do. These are the basic techniques we will be using: ujjayi; kapalabhati, or the breath of fire; and alternate nostril breathing.

Even the transitions within each breath are slow, smooth, and deliberate. The duration of each phase, from inhalation to retention to exhalation, is not nearly as important as the harmonious passage from one to the other. The rhythmic beginning and ending we have created encourages the mind to stay focused and undistracted. You will become totally absorbed in the sound and quality of your breathing. The movement sequences that follow will take on a rhythm of their own and flow.

Ujjayi Breathing

The prefix *uj* means "upward" or "expanding." It connotes a sense of preeminence and power. *Jaya* means "conquest" or "success," but interestingly, it also signifies restraint. In *ujjayi* breathing, the lungs are fully expanded and the chest is thrust out as if you were a mighty conqueror. Ujjayi breathing (or smooth, conscious breathing) can increase lung capacity, open the chest, calm the nervous system, and help to distribute oxygen to the extremities. The smooth conscious (as in thoughtful or focused) breathing you will use throughout the yoga section is called ujjayi. You will apply a mild throat lock (see p. 35) as you direct the breath more efficiently to those parts of your body that require extra attention.

EXERCISE 8: UJJAYI BREATHING

Sitting on the floor in a cross-legged position, close your mouth and inhale slowly through the nose. Now, this part is a little tricky: try to partially close the back of your throat to slow down the escape of the breath through your trachea. If you've done it correctly, you will produce a sound reminiscent of Darth Vader's breathing. Inhale to a comfortable limit, and then as you exhale, continue to contract at the back of your throat so that even the exhale sounds Darth Vader–like or like the coarse hissing sound you hear when steam escapes from a radiator. You want to feel a slight pressure in the back of your nose and throat as the air moves through your nose during inhalation and exhalation. As your comfort level increases with ujjayi, try to extend the exhale so that it lasts longer than the length of your inhale. Remember that ujjayi is a strong, sturdy, thorough, consistent, and empowering breath and will help to inspire you as you move through the more challenging yoga sequences of the Method Workout. Practice 5 to 7 ujjayi breaths before moving on to kapalabhati.

Kapalabhati

Kapala means "skull" and *bhati* means "light" or "shining." We begin every workout with the kapalabhati breath because it awakens the body and enlivens the mind. Kapalabhati ("breath of fire") is a combination of short, terse inhalation and vigorous, forceful exhalation, one breath rapidly following another, with a split second of retention after each out-breath, usually done in cycles of 28 and 56. It clears the sinuses and air pathways to the lungs, warming the body and creating a feeling of exhilaration and strength.

EXERCISE 9: KAPALABHATI BREATHING

Sit on the floor either kneeling or in a comfortable cross-legged position with your hands resting on your knees, or if you would be more comfortable, sit in a chair with your arms down by your sides. Inhale deeply through your nose and exhale through your nose. In the next breath, inhale through the nose but fill your lungs only about two-thirds full. Immediately exhale with a quick blast through the nose or the mouth by contracting your abdominals sharply and deeply, and then immediately inhale again, and exhale, and so on, until you have counted ten sets of inhale/exhale. As your stamina improves, you should be able to work your way up to 28 inhale/exhales, or blasts. For your first round, on your tenth exhalation, continue exhaling until the lungs are empty, and then inhale as deeply as you can, sweeping your arms up overhead and hooking your thumbs together as you apply the three locks. Good job! Hold the breath as long as you comfortably can, and then when you can hold the breath no longer, lift the chin and, looking straight ahead, exhale and allow the arms to float back down to your sides.

Now take a few simple ujjayi breaths, and after your third or fourth ujjayi breath, begin the second round of kapalabhati. Your goal should be to complete three rounds of kapalabhati working up to 28 breaths by your final round as a warm-up before each workout session you do. Well done!

We end every workout with alternate nostril breathing, a calm, meditative breath that stills the body and quiets the mind. This is the way we establish order and equilibrium between the yin and yang of the body, fostering relaxation and clearing the mind of superfluous thoughts. In alternate nostril breathing we use the thumb and two fingers of the right hand to regulate and control the flow of breath through the nose. Inhalation and exhalation alternate between each nostril. Thus breathing coordination is developed—an even pressure and flow is established between the two sides.

EXERCISE 10: ALTERNATE NOSTRIL BREATHING

Sit cross-legged on your mat and place the back of your left hand on your left knee. With the thumb and index fingers touching, allow the middle, ring, and pinky fingers to extend gently over your knee. With your right hand held out in front of you, fold the index and middle fingers into your palm, leaving your ring, pinky finger, and thumb extended. Take an inhalation through the nose and block both nostrils by clamping the pinky and ring finger onto the left nostril and the thumb onto your right.

Hold and retain the breath for a moment and then exhale through the right nostril by releasing the thumb while continuing to hold and block the left nostril. After exhaling completely, inhale through the same (right) nostril. Block both nostrils and retain the breath for a 5 or 6 count and then exhale for a 5 or 6 count, this time through the left nostril.

Inhale again left, retain the breath, and exhale right. Inhale right, retain the breath, and exhale left.

Continue in this fashion for at least 6 to 8 breath cycles, counting to 5 or 6 each time you retain the breath and each time you exhale.

Can you feel your sinuses beginning to open? Are you beginning to feel relaxed? You have accomplished a great deal! You are ready for meditation.

2. ESTABLISHING THE NAVEL-TO-SPINE CONNECTION

Finding your abdominal contraction, or the "navel-to-spine connection," is one of the greatest challenges you will experience as you begin this program. Once mastered, however, this connection—actually the contraction of the abdominal wall (rectus abdominus)—will enable you to capitalize on all the work of the Method and will repay your efforts a thousandfold.

For athletes and dancers, the concept is second nature. It is something they have been doing their entire lives. When I took my first ballet class at age nine, one of the first things I was told was "Pull your tummy in!" After years of rigorous training in ballet class for several hours a day, I found that lifting and holding in my stomach really paid off. Pirouettes were possible! Jumps had power and spring! I was fortunate to discover at a very early age that when the abdominals are strong, so is everything else. When the center is strong, the spine arranges itself properly in a long tall line and the body develops proportionately because of correct alignment and symmetry. This is the theory upon which the entire Method rests.

So what do you do if you haven't spent the last twenty years in a leotard and tights? You begin with a little difficulty, perhaps even a little fear and trepidation. But once you make that first connection between your abdominals and your back—and I promise that you will—even the smallest connection will open the door to a growing sense of empowerment, which will enhance everything you do. The only direction you can go from there is up.

EXERCISE 11: THE NAVEL-TO-SPINE CONNECTION

Lie down on your mat with your knees bent, feet flat on the floor. (Make sure that your knees and feet are in alignment and are hip width apart.) Spread out all ten toes and press the full surface of your feet against the floor. Feel the weight of your whole body, from your head to your tailbone, against the floor.

Remain in this position and indulge yourself in a restful moment. Fully experience it the way you would a luxurious bubble bath, a great hot-oil massage, a superb glass of Italian Barolo.

But why the digression? Why take a rest? What about the navel-to-spine connection? Have we forgotten about that? The answer lies in the complement, or the flip side, of every physical lesson I teach: the joy you experience as you are contemplating and preparing for a particular outcome is as important as focusing on the pursuit, if not more so. This is the perfect moment to introduce this important tenet of my personal philosophy: Work is always more effective after some play, rest, and reflection.

After your pause, imagine that the crown of your head is reaching across the room to the far wall, as far from the center of your body as possible. With your arms at your sides and feeling the weight of them against the floor, tiptoe your fingertips, stretching and reaching them as far away from your shoulders as they can go. You should feel your muscles working at the back of your arms and in your back. Your entire back, including your shoulders, from your head down to your tailbone (with the exception of the natural curve at the back of your neck), should be flat against the floor. This position is called a "neutral spine." (For the navel-to-spine connection and all the Pilates exercises you do, you will want to feel this length in your spine, your back naturally flat as it gives in to gravity.)

In order to make certain you are relying strictly on your abdominal muscles and not involving your hip flexors or tucking your pelvis, try this simple test: Place your hands on the tops of your thighs where your legs join your torso. There you will find your hip flexors. (Say "How do you do?" if you're meeting them for the first time!) If the pelvis is relaxed you will feel a softness in that notch—the place where a slight depression forms at the junction of the thighs and torso. Now actively tuck your pelvis by curling your pubic bone up toward your face. Suddenly you will feel your hip flexors spring into action and "pop up." Feel the difference? The purpose of identifying the hip flexors is to make sure you are engaging your abdominals without tucking the pelvis.

Now inhale and feel the natural rise of your abdomen, and as you exhale, feel its natural fall. Inhale once again, but this time as you exhale and your abdomen falls, pull your navel toward your spine. Do this at the "bottom" of the exhalation, when it is easiest to access the deeper abdominal muscles. Maintain this abdominal contraction as you begin to inhale again. (You will find that it is more difficult to inhale during a contraction. You probably won't be able to inhale as much as you did when you allowed your stomach to balloon.) Continue to pull your navel to your spine as deeply as you can while you are exhaling, and if you can, draw it in a little deeper this time.

Practice this exercise about 4 to 5 times.

3. EFFORTLESS EFFORT (Command without Tension)

When you direct your energy with laserlike concentration toward a specific goal, you can achieve a far better result than if you were to use a strategy that includes forcing or straining or trying too hard—this leads to frustration and a host of negative emotions and often to injury. Apply this invaluable precept of "effortless effort" to the Method, to all the work set out before you, and not only will you become more powerful, more supple and fit, but you will gain the ability to recognize and release tension anywhere in your body.

The breathing patterns, ujjayi and kapalabhati, for example, teach you how to direct your energy to specific parts of your body. The navel-to-spine connection uses these breathing patterns to help you focus on your abdominals and nothing more. These are but a few examples of how intertwined effortless effort is with each of the other elements and how interdependent all of the essential elements of the Method are.

Effortless effort is an Eastern state of mind that asks you to step back and trust in your body's ability to perform. It is an economizing of thought and movement, a philosophy of exercise and physicality that influences the entire syllabus of the Method.

And that blessed internal peace and confidence, that acquiescentia in seipso, as Spinoza used to call it, that wells up from every part of the body of a muscularly well-trained human being, and soaks the indwelling soul of him with satisfaction, is, quite apart from every consideration of its mechanical utility, an element of spiritual hygiene of supreme significance.

—William James

Inherent in all learning is a natural timing and flow, and there is little to be gained by pushing and striving to achieve more than you are capable of at any given moment. The old cliché about "everything in moderation" came about for a reason, and in the Method, you will be able to put the thought into practice. Balance and moderation are the keys to the cultivation of energy. When you are sensitive to the flow and rhythms of your body, you will be present in the moment and you will be acting in harmony with time.

Exercises, when viewed in this context, will truly help to "center" you. Every movement emanates from the center, which is also our emotional center. When you learn the advantage of paying attention to the energy, flow, and rhythms in your exercises and see how pushing or forcing is counterproductive, you will then begin to apply this notion of "effortless effort" to the rest of your life.

When you center your attention in the moment and act in harmony with time, you experience inner peace and fulfillment. Most of us are so preoccupied with the outcome that we overlook the process, the reason we embarked on a certain path or project. The source of our inspiration becomes lost. By staying in the present, you can do less yet gain more; you create more personal power and energy. The paradox is that by focusing on the process, you actually have a greater influence over the outcome. You can never "overdo" the work. You are always in command, in charge of the quality of your performance.

When you do the exercises in the Method, you should feel that you are directing your energies toward a specific goal, engaging your muscles with focus and smooth control. You should never feel yourself straining or pushing to execute the movements. Each exercise is designed to stretch and strengthen muscles and to open the joints and release tension. If you are able to stay in the moment, to stay with your body, with yourself, feeling the sensations your body experiences and listening to the signals your body sends to your brain, this is exactly what you can expect—greater flexibility in body and mind.

Stand or sit comfortably and clasp your palms in front of your chest. Squeeze your hands together as hard as you can—with all your might. Hold the position for at least thirty seconds and then release.

Do you think this was an example of muscle control?

Or was it muscular exertion without a whole lot of control? Chances are good that many more muscles were called into the fray than were necessary. Your shoulders were probably bunched up near your ears, your facial muscles contorted into a grimace. Even your back may have been hunched forward. Had you focused your energy and economized your movement, you would have been able to use the same amount of energy with a superior result.

Did you think about breathing? Or your center? Did you think about combining the three elements: the breath, the navel-to-spine connection, effortless effort?

Clasp your palms in front of you once again, and this time I would like you to inhale before you squeeze them together. As you exhale, draw your navel to your spine, reach the crown of your head toward the ceiling, open your shoulders down and back, and then squ-e-e-e-ze your palms together. Not with all your might but with a clear, laser-beam focus. This time the true source of your effort and energy emanated from your center. Congratulations! You have just successfully combined at least four of the Essential Elements!

4. THE PRINCIPLE OF OPPOSITION

The principle of opposition means creating an equal and opposing isometric resistance—a self-imposed resistance as opposed to a machine's, using muscles with intention and stretching them to their utmost in diametrically opposite directions.

Would it really be so wonderful if your body could reshape itself merely by "going through the motions" or by simply wishing it were so? When you

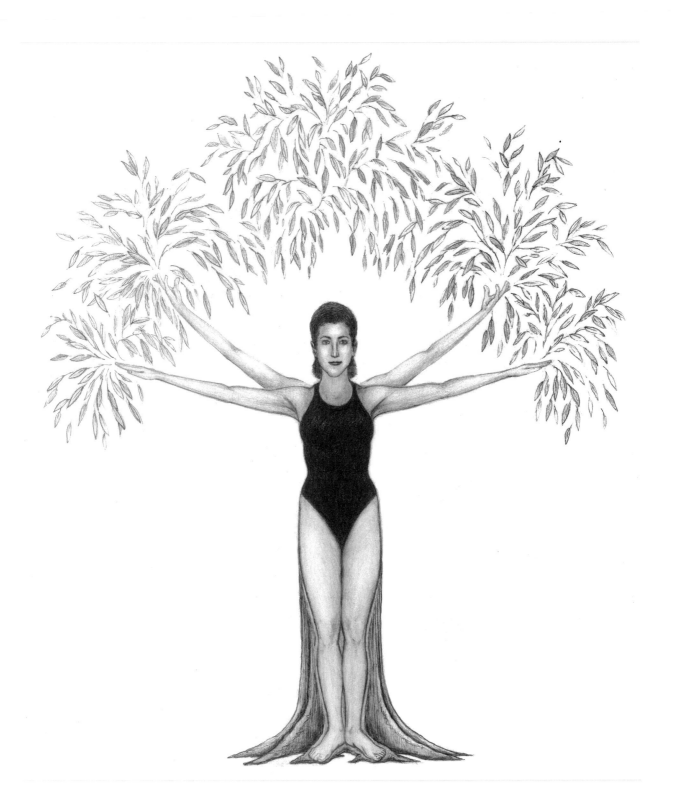

perform a movement and you do it by rote, or do it in a way that lacks enthusiasm, you are cheating yourself. If these wishes of yours could come true, not only would you be depriving yourself of the pure pleasure that comes from the experience of lengthening and strengthening simultaneously, but you would be robbing yourself of the chance to truly expand and grow. The Method alone offers the opportunity to infuse your workouts with your own flair and style, to see the desire and determination you bring to your workout reflected and mirrored in the way you move through life.

EXERCISE 13: CREATING OPPOSITIONAL RESISTANCE

Stand up straight and tall . . . a little taller, please! Reach the crown of your head toward the ceiling as high as it will go. (Imagine you are a barber shop pole spiraling upward.) At the same time, feel as if your feet were grounded to the floor, actually, pulled into the floor the way roots anchor a tree to the earth. Reach your arms up and out to your sides, fingertips extended to their utmost, and try to touch both sides of the room at once. Can you feel the muscles in your arms and back working hard to support this reaching sensation? I know you will be surprised to discover how quickly your muscles fatigue if you hold this position even for a few moments. Imagine how these few moments translate into toning time for your new body! You tone and shape your body immediately when you reach in opposite directions with focused effort.

Now reach your hand out in front of you, pointing your finger, but do it halfheartedly. Now really reach your arm out in front of you as though you were reaching for something you really wanted or needed, or as if you were trying to make a point. (Pretend you are the evil queen and you are sending Snow White up to her room. Reach your arm like that.) When you use intention as you are executing a movement, the muscles of that part of the body develop in testament to that intention. All of your muscles reflect your effort and intention. *When you stretch any part of your body, really stretch it, and then feel and observe the results. "Stretch it like you mean it!" I always tell my students.*

5. QUALITY VERSUS QUANTITY

"Much less is more," is an important part of the Method philosophy. A low number of repetitions for each of many exercises means that muscles are strengthened without creating bulk. The concentration and focus you bring to each exercise increase the quality of movement and coordination. We are led to believe that if we repeat and repeat, we strengthen and tone and shape, but what if we are aimlessly following an instructor, using our headphones as we lift weights or cycle or run or climb? What happens then? Not as much as when you concentrate and use your mind and your body. It's human nature to want to repeat something over and over in order to reach a particular goal. But doing more and more of something that is just partially effective in the first place can never compete with doing something correctly an appropriate number of times.

6. INTUITIVE INTEGRATION

Seeing the whole as a combination of component parts is the work of the conscious mind. As human beings, that's what we do. People tend to view the human form not as an entirety but broken down into anatomical structures, subdivided all the way down the chain to its cells and their DNA.

Matters of health and well-being have come to be viewed in this same compartmentalized fashion. Even the mind and the body have been separated and isolated from one another. It's as if we were a walking set of autonomous bones, muscles, nerves, and blood vessels, each wanting and needing to be attended to, each with an agenda of its own.

This same philosophy is mistakenly applied to exercise. We tend to work on certain parts of the body, actually believing we can separate them from the rest. No matter how we focus on one part of our body with our conscious mind, we find that the part we have chosen to isolate exists and functions only in connection with the whole. The whole fades into the background when we focus on just one aspect, but the whole still exists.

In this same sense, just the collection of parts does not produce a whole. Often a physical problem appears only in one part of the body and people get the impression that this is the only part that has a problem, but a problem actually exists in the body as a whole. Everything in your body is connected. Our conscious mind is effective in distinguishing parts and defining their role as a means to understanding the whole. Our mind can therefore be applied to create a higher order of integration. "Integrated isolations," or points of focus, are moments in time, as during the Single-Leg Pull, for example, during which, although you are focusing on a rather large movement combination—pulling one knee in while stretching the other leg out straight—you are at the same time concentrating on pulling the navel to the spine while simultaneously devoting focused attention to stretching the foot of the extended leg farther away from the body. This is an integrated isolation: isolating focus and directing effort toward not one body part but several at the same time. I have already said a number of times that working the body as an integrated whole is the most efficient way to build stamina, as opposed to isolating specific body parts. All the components in the Method adhere to this philosophy. We need to learn with our entire being, not just body, not just mind. When you practice the Essential Elements and the various exercises of the Method, experience them! Your whole self will feel them and inform you. Practice and repeat them as many times as you need to in order to feel a growing sense of confidence not only in the execution of the movements but, more importantly, in yourself.

EXERCISE 14: QUALITY AND QUANTITY WITH INTUITIVE INTEGRATION

Sitting right there in your chair, lift your right knee to your chest. Lift it 20 times up and down if you can and don't give a second thought to form or posture. How was that? You will probably feel the muscles in your thighs and in your hip flexors, and you will definitely feel that it was grunt work. You will have succeeded in fatiguing the muscles used, but where was the form? Your posture? The attention to detail? The economy of movement, combined with the focus of the breath, directing your efforts to important elements such as the principle of opposition and the navel-to-spine connection?

Now then, let's try that again, and you are only going to lift your knee to your chest 10 times, and believe me, you will feel the muscles in your leg more deeply, more completely than you ever thought possible.

Sitting up tall, reaching the crown of your head to the ceiling and pulling the navel to the spine to establish perfect posture, inhale, and as you exhale, lift your knee to your chest as high as you can. Hold it there for a 3-count and then lower it with control. Make sure you don't slump forward but that you use your abdominals to help lift the leg. (Now you're working your abs too, an example of intuitive integration coming up.) Now, even after the fourth or fifth repetition, you are feeling your leg, almost feeling the inner workings of the muscles themselves and the interdependent workings of the body as it functions optimally as an integrated whole. With focused attention, body and mind working together, less is definitely more!

7. TRANSITIONS—JUST AS IMPORTANT AS THE EXERCISES THEMSELVES

The Method Workout is like a carefully choreographed dance designed in such a way that even the moments between each exercise can further enhance your workout.

If you maintain your concentration and control for the entire 30 to 45 minutes of your sessions, if you dedicate yourself, and I mean for every single minute, not only will you develop a sense of athleticism, but you will tone, lengthen, and strengthen your body at the same time. You will see results quickly.

Treat each moment between your exercises as a golden opportunity to further enhance your practice. If you can remain as intentional during the transitions as you are when you do the core movements, you will truly learn how to hone your skills and appreciate the difference between work and rest, and you will be able to bask in the sunshine of your efforts. Before you know it, you will experience a seamlessness in your regime, like a stream of consciousness that affords you the opportunity to evolve, becoming more and more precise, stronger, more graceful, more fit each time you do it. I promise you will glory in the rewards.

EXERCISE 15: TRANSITIONS

From a sitting position on your chair, your couch, or your bed, stand up, and as you do, use the navel-to-spine connection. That's right! Reach the crown of your head toward the ceiling and place your feet firmly against the floor (the principle of opposition). As you stand up, inhale, and begin your exhale as you return to a sitting position, using the navel-to-spine connection just as you did when you stood up so gracefully. Instead of collapsing or slumping back into your chair or onto your bed, do you see that you were maintaining the thread of control in your body? You held your focus and as a result moved elegantly and efficiently. Even when you are getting ready to relax, you use the core muscles of your body. This is how you will move from exercise to exercise in your Method workout.

8. TEMPO AND DYNAMIC

Tempo and dynamic are the way you start to see results quickly. In order for your muscles to be sufficiently challenged and entirely supple, strong, and responsive, they need to experience a full spectrum of tempos. If you were always to move at one tempo, your muscles would only know that one way to move and when challenged with an alternative rhythm would be at a loss, would not be "up to speed," in essence.

Think for a moment that you want to view your body as you would a car. If you were in the market for a new car, you would take it for a test drive and take all the details into account: a strong pickup, smooth handling and control, a kind of effortless command, power, sturdy brakes, and so on. In the Method you will discover a full spectrum of tempos, so that the muscles of your body, like the car you would choose, will be well versed (flexible in every range of motion) and demonstrate capability in every kind of dynamic, from slow, steady, legato movements that are deeper in character (for warm-up exercises intended to stretch and strengthen at a more mindful pace, such as the Roll-Up, a fairly slow and methodical exercise) to the faster, lighter, laser-beam-like stacatto motions (for the Hot Potato, for instance, a part of the Side Series, an exercise that moves quickly in order to challenge the muscle bodies differently and target specific muscles in the legs, hips, and buttocks).

You will discover that every exercise has a specific tempo geared toward producing a specific result. Your body's overall coordination and balance will improve as the individual muscles of your body learn and respond to the dynamics of different tempos and become more conditioned, responsive, and toned.

EXERCISE 16: TEMPO AND DYNAMIC

Very simply, sitting in your chair or cross-legged on the floor, lift your right arm up from the side of the body, extending it out from the shoulder, employing all the essential elements you believe you can apply to this physical moment. Imagine an adagio—slow, lyrical music—and create a movement quality that imitates the sounds you hear in your head. Lift your arm slowly as you inhale and lower it slowly with control as you exhale. Do this 5 times. Check in with yourself and note how the arm feels, how the core body (trunk) feels. Repeat the arm lifts with the left side for balance and symmetry. Now let's speed things up a little. Lift your right arm up and bring it down quickly, as though you were listening to the "Flight of the Bumble Bee" or something similar in tempo. Do you feel how much more effort is required to maintain the core body, to keep it still as you move your arm up and down at this new speed? You really have to pull your navel to your spine and feel the principle of opposition at work to maintain stillness in your torso and con-

centrate on moving just the arm (another example of point of focus and intu-
itive integration). Of course, you should be mindful of keeping the body still
and tall when you move either slowly or quickly. Both slow and steady and
quick and firey are tempos that tone the muscles involved and are effective as
long as you remember to focus on the body as an integrated whole.

9. MEDITATION

The mind has a strong penchant for drifting aimlessly in ever shifting seas of thought and fantasy. The Chinese Taoists call the mind a playful monkey and Indian yogis compare it to a wild horse that refuses to be tethered.

Since the "mind is the leader of energy and where the mind goes energy follows" according to *The Yellow Emperor's Classic of Internal Medicine*, if the mind is absent during breathing exercises, your body's energy has no commander and strays about aimlessly, scattering and leaking instead of gathering and circulating. At the core of the entire breathing process lies the mind.

Meditation is a time for clearing the mind of superfluous thoughts. It is a time for introspection and reflection, for calm, for peace . . . for nothingness. It takes time to learn the art of meditation. It requires dedication and practice, but it is by no means impossible. As in effortless effort, meditation happens when you are not trying at all. It happens in the absence of exertion, not in its presence. It takes time.

It is only when we silence the blaring sounds of our daily existence that we can finally hear the whispers of truth that life reveals to us, as it stands knocking on the doorsteps of our hearts.

—K. T. Jong

EXERCISE 17: MEDITATION

Sit in a comfortable cross-legged position on your mat or in your chair and close your eyes. Inhale and exhale in the ujjayi style and then begin alternate nostril breathing. Do several rounds of alternate nostril breathing, and then bring the back of your hand to rest on your right knee. Continue to breathe without effort, just natural full diaphragmatic breaths. Allow the stomach to expand and release easily.

Turn your attention and your perceptions inward. Listen to the sounds of your breath. Listen to your heartbeat. Don't allow an external sound to distract you. Energy follows the mind, so if you maintain your focus, your internal energy will gather and you will begin to feel a sense of stillness and calm.

Silence the internal dialogue. Stop talking to yourself about thoughts and feelings and give yourself over to the moment. Focus on the rhythm and the quality of your breath and you will feel lighter and more centered, more peaceful, more grounded.

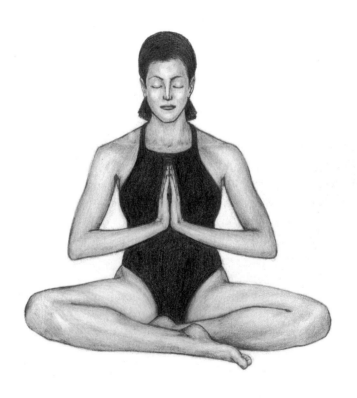

4

DIPPING YOUR FOOT IN THE POOL:

Pre-exercises

Every one of us has in him a continent of undiscovered character. Blessed is he who acts the Columbus to his own soul.
—William Habbington

I N THIS CHAPTER we'll discuss how to begin, which level (1, 2, or 3) you should follow, and the circumstances of your workout.

Try to find an area in your home where you are in harmony with your surroundings. Perhaps near a window, especially if you have one that looks out over a garden or pleasant landscape. Choose a cozy room but one that is well ventilated and not cluttered. You don't want to have to worry about knocking into anything and you'll need enough stretch-out space to be able to extend your body in all directions, with a foot or two to spare. Most of all, you want to feel comfortable and free, so choose a space that belongs to you, where you have enough room to really let loose.

As for what to wear, choose something comfortable, whatever you feel best in when you think about exercise. For some this will mean comfy sweats or shorts and for others, something more body conscious and revealing. As you progress you will probably want to wear the kind of clothing that will highlight your body's new curves, that will allow you to appreciate the beautiful sculptural changes that will be occurring from session to session. Just look at yourself in the mirror each time you work out and watch your body emerge.

Working out two or three times a week is just fine—or more (I work out every day but Sunday)—for a minimum of 30 to 45 minutes. Any time of day will do, as long as it's not on a full stomach, if you can help it. If you're fortunate enough to be able to work out at the same time every day, your workouts will become second nature to you, like brushing your teeth or combing your hair. The most exciting aspect of the Method Workout is that you will start to see results almost immediately. Most people report that after just one week of following the program, friends and family tell them they are looking taller, slimmer—and they *do* feel taller, slimmer, stronger, and more energetic.

As for equipment, all you'll need is a sticky mat for the yoga asanas (postures), a padded mat or carpet for the Pilates exercises, a sturdy chair (to be used as a ballet bar) for the dance exercises, and optionally, a light handheld pair of 3- to 5-pound weights for the Standing Sculpting Series. You can buy all these in your nearest sporting goods store. Add to these a measure of concentration, commitment, and enthusiasm and you will have provided yourself with all you require for exceptional Method workouts, now and in the future.

Finally, "Which level should I follow?" I'm certain you'll find that to be a simple matter as well. The workouts of the Method build progressively and cumulatively, and I have divided them into three levels. *Each level is a complete and effective full-body workout.* To get started all you have to do is take this simple placement test to find out which level best suits your needs and where you should begin. Then, in chapter 5, you will find all the Method Workout exercises designated as appropriate for level 1, 2, or 3, and you will design your own workout to suit your own level of capability.

EVALUATION/PLACEMENT TEST (Can You Do a Pre-Roll-Up without Moving Your Feet?)

We're going to do an exercise called the Pre–Roll-Up. How well you do this roll-up will determine at what level—1, 2, or 3—you begin the Method Workout (to see a Pre–Roll-Up, go to page 100). It's as simple as that!

Here we go: the Pre–Roll-Up:

Lie on your back, with knees bent and feet flat and your upper body relaxed into the floor. Extend your arms above your head and about 3 inches off the floor. Inhale, *and as you* exhale, *begin to reach your fingertips up toward the ceiling, and in a continuous arc,* reach *your fingertips toward your knees,* peeling *your upper body* up and off *the floor and as close to sitting up as you can* without *moving your feet. How did you do? Which one of the following describes* you? *(To accurately test your abdominal strength, you should do the exercise slowly and not cheat by using momentum in order to get all the way up off the floor in one motion.)*

Begin at level 1 *if you started to roll up and got stuck pretty much at the beginning. Your shoulder blades were just starting to come up off the floor but you couldn't get too much farther and needed to use your hands—you may even have tried placing your hands behind your thighs so you could pull yourself up the rest of the way to complete the roll-up. Even with this little bit of help, your feet began to leave the floor. If this describes you, or is close to describing you, begin at level 1.*

Begin at level 1, *as well, if you rolled up and your shoulder blades and upper body were almost completely off the floor. Your feet may have shifted slightly, but then again, maybe they didn't move at all. You may have had to use your hands behind your thighs so you could complete the roll-up. If any or all of these describe you or are close to describing you, you should follow level 1 exercises for 4 to 6 weeks and then move on to level 2.*

If you are a beginner and your placement test results direct you to level 1, plan on and feel good about staying on with level 1 for at least 2 to 3 weeks, perhaps as long as 4 to 6 weeks, and the same is true for you if you are starting on level 2. The most important thing to remember is that you want to feel comfortable and confident wherever you are, always inspired by the element of the mildly "unattainable" or the presence of challenge, which is integral to your progress.

Begin at level 2 (but do level 1 exercises the first five times you do the workout) if you were able to roll up smoothly, with control and deliberateness: if you were able to peel your upper back, middle back, and then your lower back off the floor completely. If your feet shifted or moved even a little bit during the roll-up, you should follow level 1 for 2 to 4 weeks, level 2 for 4 to 6 weeks, and then advance to level 3, or the complete Method Workout.

Begin at level 3 if you rolled up flawlessly *(but do level 1 and 2 exercises the first two times you do the workout to be certain you are fully prepared for level 3).*

Remember, each level is a complete and effective full-body workout. What is most important, therefore, is *not* what your recommended level is or what you are currently working on but how *comfortable and capable* you feel while you are doing each exercise.

Let's use level 1 as an example: On a typical day you begin with pre-exercises (more about this in a moment), the warm-up that will prepare your body and familiarize you with the exercises in the workouts for all levels. Then one by one you do the individual exercises that make up the body of work for the level 1 workout. Follow this routine for 4 to 6 weeks, 2 to 3 times per week, for 30- to 45-minute sessions, and you will begin to develop a competency and skill in performing them. As soon as you feel you can complete all these exercises with *comfort and ease* and you need a greater challenge, simply add an exercise, one or two at a time, from level 2, or whichever level is one higher than your present one.

As you progress and have combined all the exercises from level 1 with level 2, add an exercise, one or two at a time, from level 3, until you are doing the complete Method Workout.

Do you ever discard an exercise after you feel you have mastered it? That's a good question, but I think you already know the answer. You refine and re-refine every exercise. You add and accumulate, master and refine, until you are doing more and more, and before you know it *all* the exercises from level 1 and level 2 join the growing list and become your very own complete Method Workout.

THE PRE-EXERCISES

Before you begin the pre-exercises, you may want to consult the Appendix. You will find a helpful, thought-provoking questionnaire, providing you with information on self-evaluation. The Appendix questionnaire is a nice way to acquaint yourself with your body and its capabilities in much the same way a trainer would when first meeting you. Take your time as you answer the questions. They will help you figure out where to begin.

Even if you passed the placement test with flying colors, I recommend that you take full advantage of the series of exercises I call pre-exercises. Use them to prepare and warm up your body for whichever level of workout you are doing.

Just as scales and arpeggios are the bricks and mortar for musicians and vocalists, the pre-exercises will provide you with a foundation for all the work that lies ahead. Not only will they increase your overall strength and coordination, but because they are simple and uncomplicated, mastering them will boost your confidence right at the outset and heighten your ability to take on greater challenges as you train. This is the first time of many times when I will ask you to leave your readerly mind behind and just try things. Experiment physically!

The following are the six pre-exercises:

No. 1: Dipping Your Foot in the Pool
No. 2: Head Lift
No. 3: Point of Control
No. 4: Standing Positions
No. 5: Point, Flex, and Lengthen
No. 6: Campfire Breathing

Don't be afraid to give your best to what seemingly are small jobs. Every time you conquer one it makes you that much stronger. If you do the little jobs well, the big ones will tend to take care of themselves.

—Dale Carnegie

NO. 1: DIPPING YOUR FOOT IN THE POOL

This is an important pre-exercise, one you should do at the beginning of every session for the first 2 or 3 weeks. It will prepare you for the level 1 and level 2 workouts, zeroing in on your core muscles and your navel-to-spine connection.

1. *Lying down on your back with the knees bent and feet flat on the floor aligned with your knees, extend your arms long and press them against the floor. Feel your body sinking into the floor.*
2. *Inhale, and at the bottom of the exhalation (meaning when your lungs are completely empty), lift the right knee toward your chest without shifting the hips or moving the pelvis. Inhale, and as you exhale, lower the right foot back down to the floor.*
3. *Switch to the left side. Inhale, and when you have emptied the lungs completely, find the navel-to-spine connection (remember?) and draw the left knee to the chest. Inhale, and at the bottom of the exhalation, lower the left foot to the floor with control.*
4. *Inhale and exhale, and at the bottom of the exhalation, without changing your neutral spine position (the natural lower lumbar curve of the spine against the floor), and without tucking the pelvis excessively or hunching or distorting the position of the upper back against the floor, draw both knees in toward the chest, pressing the backs of the arms against the floor.*
5. *Inhale, and at the bottom of the exhalation, lower the knees toward the floor, returning the feet to their starting position, all the while continuing to maintain the navel-to-spine connection, keeping the lower back anchored to the floor without tucking the pelvis excessively.*

NO. 2: HEAD LIFT, OR "EYES ON YOUR BELLY BUTTON"

When you lie on your back in preparation for the Pilates exercises of the Method Workout, if your head is positioned properly you should be able to see your belly button when you raise your head up off the mat. Your chin should curl toward your chest but not press against it, because this would cause unnecessary strain on the muscles of the neck and upper back.

As a beginner, your neck may tire easily, and until your core is sufficiently developed, your neck muscles will probably overcompensate. So if you are not able to execute the exercises with comfort and ease and your neck feels excessively tired or strained, please put your head down, and when you do, know that as you gain strength your comfort level will increase and eventually you won't be aware of your neck at all. Practice lifting your head up off the mat in preparation for the Hundred and other Pilates exercises to come:

1. *Lying on your back in the exact position you were in when you began the pre-exercise Dipping Your Foot in the Pool—your head is down, knees are bent, feet and back are flat on the floor (feet just below and aligned with your knees)—feel the length of the backs of your arms along the floor, the weight of your body anchored to the floor.*
2. *Inhale, and as you exhale, lift the head so your chin is about 2 inches above your chest and your eyes are focused on your belly button.*
3. *Stay right there. As you exhale and inhale a second time, remember to keep the navel to the spine.*
4. *As you begin to exhale again, lower your head back down to the floor, and then repeat. Inhale (while your head is still down on the floor), and on the exhale, lift the head up, eyes on the belly button, and this time make sure that your shoulders feel broad and as relaxed and uninvolved as possible. (Imagine that the backs of your shoulders are held down to the floor with Velcro.)*
5. *In the head-lift position it's natural for your shoulders to lift up a little, just as long as the bottoms of your shoulder blades are in contact with the floor and you are not experiencing excessive tightness or fatiguing in the shoulder region.*
6. *Perform the head lift 5 to 7 times, or until you are doing it with comfort and ease. Each time after that try to hold the position for at least one breath more. For example, inhale (with head down), and exhale as you curl your chin to your chest. Stay there! Contracting the abdominals as*

you inhale, exhale and inhale again. On the next exhale, lower your head back down to the floor. The next time you do the head lift, try to stay up there for 3 whole breaths. Exhale as you curl the chin up, then inhale and exhale, inhale and exhale, inhale and exhale, inhale, and then lower your head to the floor.

7. *This is the way we develop the muscular stamina you'll need in preparation for the Hundred. When you do the Hundred, you're going to keep your head lifted while you do—that's right—one hundred breaths.*

NO. 3 : POINT OF CONTROL

One of the most important things you need to consider when starting the Pilates exercises of the Method Workout is the angle at which you will work your legs, because that angle, your point of control, will ensure the safety of your back and help you strengthen and tone your abdominals more effectively.

1. *Lying on your back, drawing both knees in to the chest as you did for Dipping Your Foot in the Pool, place your arms down by your sides.*

2. *With the spine long, extend your legs up toward the ceiling, making the legs as straight as possible by engaging the quadriceps (the front of the thigh). Note that if, when you attempt this, you feel even the slightest strain or stress or worrisome discomfort in your upper back, your lower back, or your neck, you should bend your knees. As you extend your legs upward, keep them in this bent-knee position every time you attempt this pre-exercise until you develop the strength in your abdominals to support the full extension of your legs.*

3. *On the other hand, if you feel fine, try to draw the kneecaps up, or straighten the knees when your legs are extended (this will stretch the hamstrings, something you will learn more about when you discover my "InSight" about muscle pairings later in this chapter), and then inhale.*

4. *As you exhale, lengthen and lower your extended legs down straight in front of you until you have reached that "certain angle" to the floor, your*

point of control, the position you can hold while your back remains flat and your abdominals are contracted and working hard.

Position your legs at this angle for all the Pilates exercises that call for your point of control, until, after a few weeks of practice and increased strength and stamina, you will be able to lower your legs even closer to the floor. You will know when you are ready for this, because you will have a sense of comfort and ease with all the exercises. You will be progressing.

When you are satisfied that you have found "your" angle, or point of control, try to maximize or make the most of the movement by incorporating an old friend, an Essential Element called the principle of opposition: Feel as though your toes are trying to reach so far away from your core that they can actually touch the top of the wall in front of you. At the same time, feel the crown of your head spiraling out and away toward the wall behind you.

By using the principle of opposition you can create an effect of virtual weightlessness in your legs. This is not to say that you won't feel them hanging out there in front of you, or that you won't have to be working quite hard to support them, but by reaching the legs in the opposite direction from your head, you will be connecting the legs to the abdominals to create greater support for your back and thus, not only will your work be a great deal easier, but you will be creating the long, lean muscles in your legs that Pilates made famous.

NO. 4: STANDING POSITIONS: THE FOOT AND LEG STANCE FOR STANDING, SIDE-LYING, PRONE, AND SUPINE POSITIONS IN PILATES, YOGA, AND DANCE

Tripod, Parallel, and Turned Out

Three positions we will be using throughout the Method are tripod (Pilates), parallel (yoga), and turned out (dance). In each instance your objective will be to establish proper posture. Try, if possible, to position yourself in front of a mirror so you can check your alignment and see what a difference just a few changes in your carriage will make.

Tripod: Heels Together, Toes Apart

This position is used in many of the exercises and may be taken while you are lying on your back (supine positions), on your side (Side Series), or on your stomach (prone positions), as well as when you are standing for the Standing Sculpting Series.

1. *Standing upright, feet in a parallel position, rock back on your heels so that there is little weight remaining on the balls of your feet.*
2. *In one motion, with heels together, open your feet so they form a "tripod," not too wide and not too narrow. The distance between your big toes should be approximately 4 to 6 inches.*
3. *Squeeze your inner thighs together and lift the fronts of the thighs so your legs feel long and straight.*
4. *Squeeze your buttocks as you clasp your hands behind your back, and as you draw your clasped hands and arms down behind you a bit farther (which will open the shoulders naturally), lengthen the neck and lift the crown of the head toward the ceiling, in opposition to your lengthened legs.*
5. *Open the chest and lift your eyes slightly above the horizon so you are standing tall and proud.*
6. *Translate this very tall, proud, long feeling to every Pilates exercise you do, whether you are lying on your back, stomach, or side or are standing. You will look and feel taller.*

Parallel: Heels and Toes Together

Aside from the postural benefits of this position, you will actually be using the parallel stance in *all* your yoga poses, whether it be sitting, standing, or lying down, whether the feet are touching or are separated by a considerable distance. In almost all the yoga asanas, some of the Pilates exercises, and a few of the dance exercises, your feet will assume this parallel stance.

1. *Standing tall once again, bring your feet together, with your big toes touching and your heels in line.*

2. *Feel the full surface of the foot against the floor and draw the inner thighs together without changing the placement of your legs as they extend down from your hips.*

3. *Draw your kneecaps up by engaging the quadriceps (fronts of your thighs) and squeeze the gluteals (buttocks) together so that the pelvis tucks under ever so slightly, which brings your pubic bone up, as opposed to its being tipped slightly downward in its resting state.*

4. *Open your chest, shoulders down and back, and feel the crown of your head spiraling up toward the ceiling.*

5. *Feel the strength in this pose, which is also called Mountain Pose in yoga. Feel like a tall, sturdy mountain, with your head reaching up into the clouds and your feet grounded into the layers of rock that lie below.*

Turned Out: Heels Together and Toes Wide Apart

In classical ballet, "turned out" is the position used for every movement, one in which the legs are externally rotated in the hip sockets. In using this position we tone the gluteus medius and minimus and the piriformis, and the abductors and rotators of the upper legs, firming and shaping the muscles of the hips and buttocks in a slightly different way than in the parallel position, where we tend to strengthen the adductors, or inner thighs.

1. Standing tall, *bring your feet together, with your big toes touching and heels in line in a parallel position as you did in the previous exercise.*

2. Rock back *onto your heels so that there is little weight remaining on the balls of your feet, and in one swift, though carefully controlled, motion, open the toes so they come to rest about 6 to 8 inches apart, which is a bit wider than we used in establishing the tripod stance.*

3. *When establishing your turn-out, it is very important that you respect your body's natural range of motion in the hips and that you never force your turn-out past a comfortable line of rotation, or a 50- to 65-degree angle.*

4. Working from the floor up, *draw your legs together, squeezing your inner*

thighs and engaging the quadriceps to complete a long, tall, fully extended line through the legs. (Your knees should be lined up over your toes.)

5. *The buttocks should be tight and your spine should feel tall from your tailbone all the way up and through to the crown of your head.*

6. *We will use the turned-out position (or first position) for all the ballet exercises, which you will find toward the end of the Method Workout.*

NO. 5: POINT, FLEX, AND LENGTHEN, OR "THREE FOOT POSITIONS THAT ARE MORE IMPORTANT THAN YOU THINK!"

The Long, Loosely Pointed Foot

For most of the Pilates exercises you want to use a long, loosely pointed foot, not a foot that is flexed or pointed hard (unless specified). When you are asked to extend through a soft point, or long, loosely pointed foot, your foot is not literally slack or soft but instead is directed, but gently, toward a point of focus away from the center of the body (incorporating the principle of opposition).

The soft point, or long, loosely pointed foot, works the muscles of the upper leg and gluteals, toning and sculpting the upper leg, hips, and buttocks while conditioning and strengthening the muscles of the foot for those times when you need to strongly point or flex it.

You can practice the long, loosely pointed foot while sitting right where you are:

Stretch your big toe toward a point on the wall and allow the rest of your foot to follow. Feel that you are stretching the foot with the help of the entire leg.

Reach with it and you will be able to feel that "reach" extending all the way up and into your upper leg, all the way through to your core. (This is what is meant by the phrase lengthening through.)

Suddenly you will feel there is life in your leg and you've lengthened and strengthened the whole side of your body. By virtue of reaching one loosely pointed foot you are conditioning an entire length of connective tissue and muscles, all the way down to your bones.

Now repeat this "physical moment" on the opposite side for symmetry and balance, and since we all have both a dominant and a weaker side to our bodies, see how the level of strength and coordination differs from side to side.

Once you acknowledge the differing capabilities of each side of your body and embrace the differences, once you have introduced the two sides of your body to one another, your ability to cultivate a more balanced, symmetrical, and functional body increases significantly. A balanced body has far greater potential for overall strength, in all ranges of motion; has increased natural defense against injury; and is more supple, more agile, and more capable.

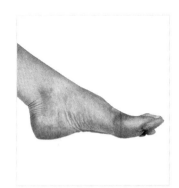

Flexing the Foot, or "Look at the Heels on Your Shoes!"

Flexing the foot is easy enough when you do it casually or without intention, but when you flex the foot in the Method Workout, think about flexing the foot plus all five toes.

Once you learn to flex your foot correctly, as you will in the pre-exercise ahead, not only will you strengthen the muscles in your feet and create proper alignment, but you will balance your gait and walk more efficiently, actually realigning and reeducating your whole body posture in a musculoskeletal sense.

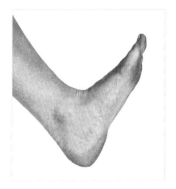

Let's try a simple experiment:

1. *Flex your foot by bringing all five toes back toward your leg, flexing them toward your shin as symmetrically as you can.*
2. *Now flex your foot as you would naturally (meaning without trying to do anything in particular with the toes, just letting them flex without any special effort or focus). Observe what happens as opposed to when you flexed it symmetrically in direction 1 when you were concentrating on something specific.*

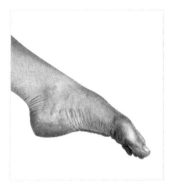

When you flexed your foot the second time, did the big-toe side of your foot do most of the work? Did it show a greater range of motion? Or was the baby-toe side easier to pull back? For most of us, the big-toe side is the runaway winner (you knew that!), and it is the outer edge, or the baby-toe side, that seems always to require more attention and strengthening.

Let's take a moment so you can familiarize yourself with the flexed position:

1. *Lift your leg out in front of you as you sit in your chair and extend the foot so it is an extension of the leg.*
2. *Inhale, and then as you exhale, flex the foot toward you, then inhale as you point it away (in a relaxed counter-, or opposite, movement to the flex).*
3. *As you exhale, flex the foot toward you again and hold the flexed position for a few seconds. Repeat this exercise 5 to 7 times on each foot before you move on.*

The Hard Point, or "Why Should You Point Your Foot Like a Ballerina If You're Never Going to Wear a Tutu?"

If you are asked to "point the foot" in any of the Method exercises, lengthen and curl it into a curved position and direct your focus and energy in one long continuous line all the way down your leg to the tip of your big toe.

You don't want to sacrifice form by pointing it too hard. Remember the concept of effortless effort? Unless you are a dancer and have spent years developing the intricate network of muscles in the foot, be reminded that even the most athletic, conditioned, and disciplined bodies will experience foot cramping when asked to point a foot in this manner for the first time.

Most people don't pay any attention to the foot, so the muscles are unprepared to honor special requests. In the Method Workout, every single muscle is used, and as a result you strengthen your entire body from

THE BENEFITS OF EQUILIBRIUM

Have you ever looked at the sole of your shoe and noticed that one side of the heel is worn down? That is usually a clear indication that one part of your foot is mechanically dominant and the other is underutilized. Creating an equilibrium with your foot alignment is a model for the rest of your body and will show you how the exercises truly form a bridge between your exercise hours and improving the quality of the rest of your life. When you experience an ache or a pain in your upper back, or in your shoulder, the last thing you would consider is the idea that perhaps this ache or pain was caused by an imbalance in your gait, which in turn affected your hip placement, which then influenced the way you held your back to compensate. The unbelievable truth is that many aches and pains are caused by structural imbalances in the body that start way down there with your feet. Imagine! You can often actually realign your body by starting with your feet and working your way up to the crown of your head. Convincing your body to let go of habits is no easy task. Your body knows what it knows and is extraordinarily faithful to familiar pathways and patterns, but with practice and repetition of a new, more promising set of stimuli, you'll be left feeling conditioned and invigorated. The exercises of the Method reward the body and the mind constantly, encouraging you in an almost subliminal fashion to release outmoded ways of thinking and working with your body. Retraining your body and gently suggesting that it allow old useless habits to die is entirely possible once you see and feel a difference after investing your time in a pursuit that yields such rich rewards. Even if you suffer from scoliosis (curvature of the spine) or chronic idiopathic pain (without a clear source or cause), you can truly hope to rehabilitate yourself by paying careful attention to each and every part of your body and by observing how each part contributes to the integrated whole by examining each individual role and the function it serves when the body moves synergistically.

Since creating a new balance between the two sides of the foot can impact the entire body, when you are asked to flex the foot in the Pilates and yoga exercises, flex the baby-toe side back toward your shin as much as or *even a bit more than* the big-toe side. Not only will you foster better foot alignment and begin to establish "fairness," or equilibrium, between the two outer edges, but you will be strengthening the entire foot, preparing it for standing, walking, and running, and creating a broader, more even surface for the standing poses and all the other exercises you do.

the crown of your head all the way down to your baby toe. But like the abdominals, feet require time and practice in order to develop the kind of functional, integrative strength inherent in the Method Workout.

The other reason the feet cramp is that proper breathing is often ignored when you are asked to perform a new and challenging movement. The brain is so busy that, in this case, the foot is deprived of its fair share of oxygen. Direct your attention to the breath; actually send your breath to your foot as you point it, and chances are that it will not cramp. If it should, it won't remain in a cramp for long but will release and assume its intended position, the "point" you are striving for.

The best way to practice pointing your foot is by brushing it along the floor, actually using the floor as leverage.

1. *Stand and hold on to the back of a chair, pulling the navel to the spine (as always). Stand in the turned-out position, as we learned in the previous pre-exercise.*
2. *With your feet in this position and pulling your navel to the spine (as always),* brush *the big toe of your right foot, with laser-beam focus and a substantial amount of effort, toward a point on the floor in front of you, down the midline of your body. Use your big toe as the leader of your other toes in this reaching movement.*

At first your foot will probably cramp in this position. Don't try to force your way through the cramp but heed your body and rest, then breathe. Send your breath to your pointed foot (as you did with your flexed foot in the last exercise), and once the cramp or spasm subsides, try the movement again.

3. *Return the right foot back to meet the left (in its original turned-out position) and brush it in the same manner you used when you brushed it forward, but in reverse. Lead with the baby-toe side of the foot, bringing it toward the standing leg, "allowing" the big toe to join.*
4. *Then release the ball of the foot into the floor, then the arch, until the full*

surface of the foot is resting flat against the floor, supporting the body in a turned-out position.

Repeat the hard point 4 to 6 times with the right foot and then switch and repeat 4 to 6 times with the left.

You just learned how to do a tendu. Your very first ballet exercise with me!

NO. 6 CAMPFIRE BREATHING, OR SEATED PREPARATION FOR THE HUNDRED BREATH

I devised Campfire Breathing several years ago when I needed a more accessible, more comfortable way to teach the breathing used in the Hundred, one of the first Pilates exercises you are going to learn in level 1. Every exercise in the Method is like an onion—multilayered, and endlessly interesting as a result. But that multifaceted aspect charges me with an even greater imperative, and that is to start you out as simply as possible.

So let us begin with the breath of the Hundred all by itself. You can learn it while you are sitting around a campfire listening to some good stories, the only difference being that at our campfire you won't be toasting any marshmallows and you will have to give some of your attention to posture.

1. *Sitting upright on the floor or your mat, with your knees bent, your arms encircling your knees, lift your spine, using your arms to leverage the lift, as tall as your spine can take you (remember the barber shop pole from the Nine Essential Elements?).*
2. *Inhale, and as you exhale, pull the navel to the spine and grow even taller.*
3. *Inhale in short, terse, staccato breaths (similar to kapalabhati) 5 times, and without pausing, exhale 5 times in the same style.*
4. *Continue as seamlessly as possible, inhale 5 times, 1, 2, 3, 4, 5, and exhale 5 times, 1, 2, 3, 4, 5, challenging yourself as you inhale the fourth and fifth times because your lungs will not be accustomed to taking in so much air while maintaining a flat abdominal wall.*

5. *"Breathe in for 5 and out for 5," "in for 5, out for 5," without pause until you have completed 100 breaths, or ten times ten.*

INSIGHTS

The InSights are meant to further your understanding of one of the more technical aspects of a workout or series of exercises. They are intended to help you understand the body's dynamic, the brilliance of the workings of the body as "machine."

InSights are my secrets, my hard-won knowledge, my experience, my gift—and I will share them all with you, sprinkling them like golden fairy dust on any intricate or complicated moment that can be unraveled or understood only as if by magic. And just as Cinderella's godmother can turn any pumpkin into a royal coach, my insights will transform your every workout into its utmost possibility.

INSIGHT

Spinal Articulation

One of the most important things you will ever do is learn how to "roll through your spine" properly. Not only is it an integral component of your Method workout, but it will provide countless benefits.

Most people don't even know what good posture is, let alone how to go about establishing it. Good posture, which leads to proper musculoskeletal placement, is an added measure of positive influence that you can hope to have over your body and its myriad functions. Poor posture can cause a host of ailments, including chronic back pain, migraine headaches, poor circulation, diminished lung capacity, improper gait patterns, and general malaise.

The antidote to all of these problems is really very simple: establish good posture, thereby adopting a new muscular perception of what correct placement is for your body, and a new world of possibility will be

If you can find a path with no obstacles, it probably doesn't lead anywhere.

—Frank A. Clark

yours. Your body's musculature literally learns how to rearrange itself around a properly organized and lengthened spine, which comprises a series of natural curves. The healthy spine resembles a seahorse, or an elongated S, beginning with the cervical curve (originating at the base of the skull and coming in toward the body, resembling a soft C shape); leading into the upper back, or the thoracic length of vertebrae, which should start curving slightly outward; and then moving in to assume a long, slightly concave curve; ending finally in a lumbar curve at the low back, which slopes down and out to the sacrum, the section of your back just above your buttocks, completing itself at the coccyx, or tailbone.

Over time, through wear and tear and repetitive patterns, the configuration of the spine can lose its integrity, and the surrounding muscles, obedient and responsive (they ask no questions and support the spine's decision), rally around the new directions the spine moves in, arranging themselves into new shapes and textures, some unnaturally protruding, some disappearing from view when they should demonstrate a healthy prominence—atrophy. In the same way that the muscles of the body can be lured to "the wrong side of the tracks," they can be convinced to assume new positions that contribute to the body's mechanics and overall efficiency of movement. Reversing the effects of time is challenging but not impossible.

When you learn to move sequentially (or roll) through your spine, you massage each vertebra, along with the muscles immediately surrounding the spine. You create space between the discs in your spinal column and nourish the intervertebral sacs containing the pulp that provides the cushioning making possible the miraculous torquing, twisting, and bending movements we take for granted every day. Properly executed spinal articulation achieves the following:

1. Stretches and strengthens the spine and the muscles that surround it
2. Augments and preserves the resilience of the inner structure
3. Enhances the spine's efficiency

Physical concepts are the creation of the human mind, and are not, however it may seem, determined by our external world. In our endeavor to understand reality, we are somewhat like a man trying to understand the mechanism of a closed watch. He can see the hands move and hear its ticking, but he has no way of opening the case. If he is ingenious, he may form some picture of the mechanism which could be responsible for all the things he observes.

—Albert Einstein

Ring the bells that still can ring Forget your perfect offering. There is a crack in everything, That's how the light gets in.

—Leonard Cohen

4. Increases the spine's longevity
5. Encourages greater range of motion and overall facility in your body
6. Improves the quality of your most basic movements
7. Improves the quality of your every day

Simply by rolling through your spine (and breathing, of course), whether from a standing position or supine (the Roll-Up, for example), you can release tension and stress in the neck and shoulders and muscles of your back. *Every* exercise you will learn in the Method improves your standing posture and balances your gait pattern (the way you walk), helping you to create a machine that functions at peak efficiency in all aspects: the structural, the physiological, and the psychological.

The spine boasts its own very complicated network of neural pathways that serve as "communication highways" connecting directly to the brain. Both the sympathetic and parasympathetic nerves run along the length of the spine, along with hundreds of thousands of other nerve endings, which are forever sending their own signals to the rest of the body. When you experience stress or trauma, messages are sent from brain to body and back again, but these "feelings" do not register in the mind alone. They find "resting places" in the body, for example, lower back pain, tight hamstrings, or a stiff neck. We develop, to one extent or another, in response to the happenings in our lives, and our bodies shape themselves by mirroring these "events." Our bodies are literally the storehouses for every emotion we experience, both good and bad. Whether owing to apathy or disassociation, or through trauma and the neglect that comes as a result, muscles lose their firm, resilient capacity and atrophy; ligaments lose their elasticity; and fasciae tighten, hardening in some cases like bone. People can literally collapse under the weight of their own frustrations, anger, sadness, developing into distorted incarnations of who they once were. Or they can rise to the occasion and work with time and its challenges.

If you are in touch with yourself or you make the effort to cultivate greater sensitivity and to become more aware of the subtle connections between body and brain and develop the resources to work through difficult moments without sublimating the events that characterize them, your fasciae (connective tissue), your muscles, everything in the body from your bones down to your very cells, will respond happily to your brain's ability to do "damage control" and will become free, flexible, unfettered, pliant, agreeable. With just a small investment of your time and energy, your body will gift you with almost immediate recognition of your positive intentions, resulting in a responsiveness you may have given up on long ago.

The exercises of the Method will provide you with the tools for transformation. You can effect tremendous change in your body if you want to, and if you make the time to do it. You can learn that by cultivating self-respect, by showing yourself a little tenderness, you can create the fertile environment that fosters potential and growth. You can become your own mind-body scientist, your own private investigator, and you will be richly rewarded as you explore, for the body speaks volumes when you listen.

Let's practice spinal articulation:

1. *Standing tall, with your feet in a parallel position, hip width apart, inhale, and as you exhale, drop the chin toward the chest and let gravity take over.*
2. *Roll down sequentially through your spine: upper back, middle, and then lower back, making sure that your head and your arms are* dead *weights and that you are not creating tension in your neck and shoulders by inadvertently supporting your head.*
3. *Continue to roll down through your spine, breathing naturally and softening your knees slightly to ease tension in the lower back.*
4. *When you cannot roll down any farther, cross your arms at the elbows, bend your knees even deeper, and allow your chest and torso to fall completely onto your thighs.*
5. *Slowly, over the course of 4 or 5 breath cycles, straighten your knees to the best of your ability while maintaining the chest on the thighs and allowing the weight of your head and upper torso to pull you down toward the*

floor. In this position, feel your hamstrings and back lengthening and stretching. Breathe fully into your back and the backs of your legs. Listen to your body! If you feel any stress or strain, pull back and ease up a little—you may have gone too far. Be kind to yourself and you will safely achieve better, longer-lasting results.

6. *When you have explored your full range of motion, uncross your arms, allowing them to drop toward the floor.*

7. *Inhale, and as you exhale, start to uncurl through the spine, softening your knees and keeping your head and arms completely relaxed and fully weighted. Uncurl bone by bone up through the middle back and upper back, and finally, allow your head to return to its placement, where it floats on top of the neck and shoulders.*

8. *Standing tall, experience the full height of your frame now that you have massaged, conditioned, stretched, and lengthened your spine. Use the principle of opposition to root your feet and legs to the earth as your head spirals up toward the ceiling. Take a deep breath in and enjoy the new sensations you are feeling. Acknowledge the new energy circulating in your body.*

THE SECOND INSIGHT

Muscle Pairings

When you begin to develop a targeted set of muscles, in this case your abdominal core, other seemingly unrelated muscles feel "left out" and want to participate. They try to be "helpful," but their help is, in fact, no help at all. To the contrary, being engaging when they are not at all welcome proves to be not only a nuisance but a real detriment and a hindrance to your progress.

The Latissimus-Trapezius Connection

There is a little-known and underacknowledged antagonistic relationship between the upper trapezius muscles (traps—shoulders) and the latissimus dorsi (lats—back), which will crop up again and again throughout your Method work, particularly in the Pilates exercises, where developing the core takes center stage.

If the shoulders "raise up" to try to help you when you are attempting the Roll-Up, for example, *they* wind up doing the work your abdominals are supposed to be doing. This interferes with the very process, the *engagement of your core muscles,* the training, strengthening, and development you are trying to master.

Train yourself instead to use the muscles of your back (specifically the lats), especially when you perform the more challenging Pilates abdominal series. Not only will you begin (as a happy coincidence) to create definition in your back, but you will have found the key to progress in the Method: *building the abdominal core.*

Let's pair our insight about muscle pairings with an exercise:

Perform this exercise in front of a mirror so you can actually watch your muscles work and observe how our theory is put into practice.

1. *Sitting tall in a chair or cross-legged on your mat, lift your arms and shape them so they are in a rounded position in front of you, as though you were hugging a large balloon.*
2. *Raise your arms so they are slightly above shoulder level and see and feel your shoulders rise as well. There they go! The upper trapezius muscles are at it again, hard at work trying to lift your shoulders. And what are the latissimus dorsi muscles doing about it? Nothing.*

Here's what you can do about it:

Maintain your arms in the higher, rounded position and feel as though you were pressing the underpart of each arm onto a flat surface.

Can you feel it? Suddenly your shoulders are no longer around your ears, yet your arms are still beautifully rounded and supported. But by what? What is the magic that is holding them in place?

You may, by now, have started to become aware of your back. If you have, Bravo! Your latissimus muscles are now in action and are working in tandem with your deltoids and other muscles in your arms and back to keep the arms in place. If you were having trouble zeroing in on your lats, this next direction is especially, but not exclusively, for you:

Place your right hand about 3 to 4 inches below your left armpit, and take your left arm out to the side where it was in its rounded position.

Press your rounded arm down on that imaginary flat surface and what you will feel should astonish and delight you. Your latissimus muscle will "pop" or flair out under the touch of your hand, and this means the muscle is working.

Now look in the mirror and do this again. See how calm and relaxed the area around your left shoulder looks when your lats are engaged? The shoulder area is overworked enough as it is, with so many of us hunched in front of computers or tensed behind the wheel of a car; it should be a relief to know that you have an element of control over the matter. You can have a hand in releasing the tension in your shoulders, toning and strengthening the muscles of your back and sides, reeducating the musculature of your body.

Try one more variation just to be sure:

Take your arm out to the side in its rounded position and hold your hand on the lat area (just below your armpit). Purposely raise your left shoulder and feel how the lat goes slack when the upper trapezius (shoulder) is working?

Understanding the dynamic of this muscle pairing will maximize all your efforts in every exercise you do. That's why I tell my students it is the granddaddy of InSights.

The Quadriceps-Hamstring Connection

The muscle pairing that will significantly increase flexibility is that of the quadriceps and the hamstrings. The idea behind it is similar to but not exactly the same as the trap-lat pairing. In the case of the trap-lat pairing, by encouraging one muscle's participation, we preclude the interference of another's. However, in the quadriceps-hamstring pairing our focus is on the two muscles *alone*. We accomplish something with one muscle by disarming the other. By our engaging the quadriceps (front of the thighs), the hamstrings release and stretch. We "fool" the hamstrings into releasing and, thereby, stretching. We win the big prize in what seems like a roundabout way, and the prize is *flexibility*.

Let's take a moment to experience this muscle pairing:

1. *Lie down on your mat, establish your navel-to-spine connection, and feel both legs lengthen. Then draw the right knee to your chest and stretch your right leg to the ceiling, as close to straight up as you comfortably can.*
2. *Feel as though you were trying to reach and touch the ceiling with your big toe, so, yes, you are stretching with a long, loosely pointed foot.*
3. *Really try your best now to straighten your right knee. Challenge yourself by engaging your quadricep muscle to accomplish this. Concentrate!*

Remember: You are working the front of your thigh to stretch and gain flexibility in the back of the leg.

With the quad-hamstring connection, you can absolutely increase your flexibility. It will take some time and effort, but far less than you would imagine.

First though, check in with your upper back and neck. If you are hitching off the floor or experiencing excessive tension in these areas, be careful. You may be trying too hard (remember effortless effort), and you should probably lower the leg a bit and go at this gently:

Clasp the leg at the back of the knee or the upper thigh or at the ankle, depending upon how flexible you are. Concentrate on lengthening the leg up to the ceiling and try *not to grip the leg too hard. Remember to breathe, and breathe naturally and fully.*

Direct your breath to the back of the leg—to your hamstring, and imagine that your breath is helping the muscle relax and lengthen at the same time. (While you are breathing, continue to engage the front of the thigh.)

Feeling your thigh laboring in this way can be misleading. Don't worry about creating bulk in the leg. Because you feel the muscle fatiguing does not mean that you are overworking it. On the contrary, because you are training the muscles in your legs, using the principle of opposition as you are training, and reaching your leg as long as possible away from your core, you are creating length and strength in the muscle body—and as a result, a long, beautiful leg.

Finally, stretch it one last time! Try to pull the leg a bit closer to your torso with your hands while keeping the knee as straight as possible.
Now, switch to the other leg and begin to stretch it in the same way.

Be cognizant of which side of your body is tighter and less developed, and as you repeat this and all the exercises in the Method Workout, send some focused breath attention to the muscles on *that* side. Creating symmetry will serve as your most powerful defense against injury and bring new balance to your body.

Now, why don't you take the Pre–Roll-Up test again? Come on, try it just for fun! You'll see how much progress you've already made.

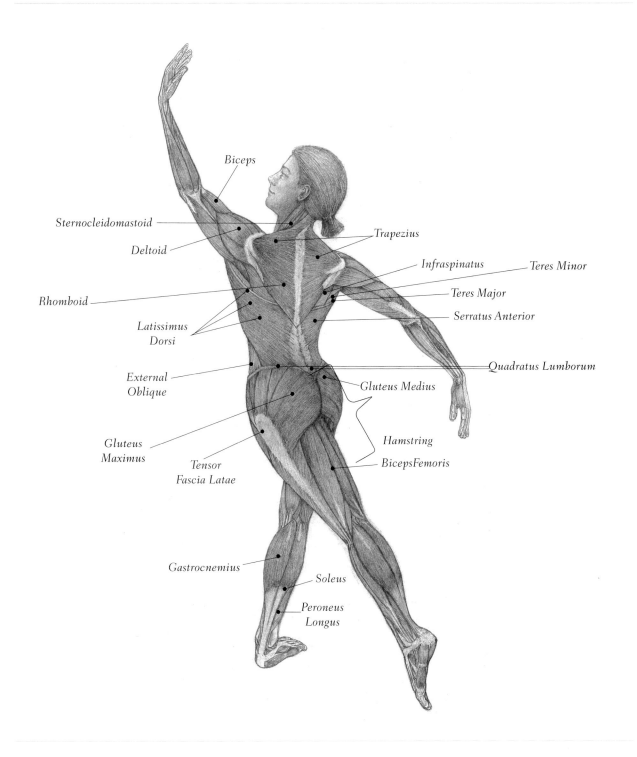

Biceps

Sternocleidomastoid

Deltoid

Trapezius

Infraspinatus

Teres Minor

Teres Major

Rhomboid

Serratus Anterior

Latissimus
Dorsi

Quadratus Lumborum

External
Oblique

Gluteus Medius

Hamstring

Gluteus
Maximus

BicepsFemoris

Tensor
Fascia Latae

Gastrocnemius

Soleus

Peroneus
Longus

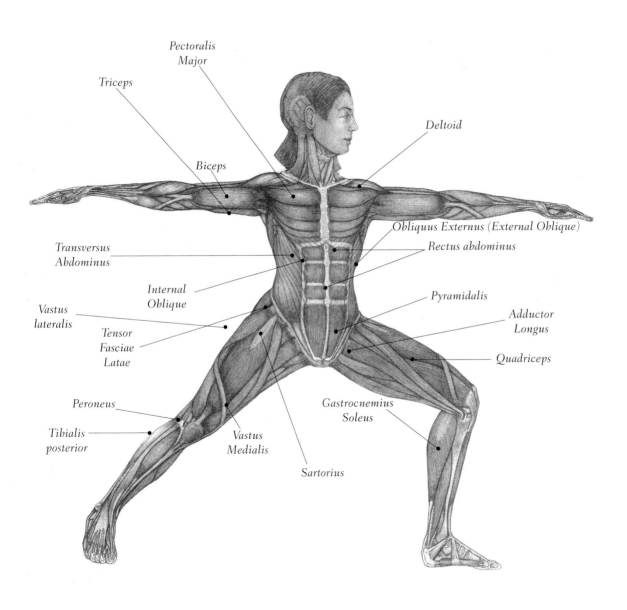

Pectoralis
Major

Triceps

Biceps

Deltoid

Obliquus Externus (External Oblique)

Transversus
Abdominus

Rectus abdominus

Internal
Oblique

Pyramidalis

Vastus
lateralis

Adductor
Longus

Tensor
Fasciae
Latae

Quadriceps

Peroneus

Gastrocnemius
Soleus

Tibialis
posterior

Vastus
Medialis

Sartorius

5

THE
METHOD
WORKOUT

There is nothing like returning to a place that remains
unchanged to find the ways in which you
yourself have altered.
—Nelson Mandela

HAVE DIVIDED Jennifer Kries' Method Workout, a selection of my own favorite exercises, into three levels. *Each level stands alone and is a complete and effective full-body workout.* You do not need to do the entire workout each time, but you certainly can. You can simply choose your favorite exercises and create a routine that lasts between 30 and 45 minutes. When you have repeated the full workout at your own level for at least 4 to 6 weeks and can complete all the exercises with *comfort and ease,* you may begin to move on to the next level. I have marked the exercises pertaining to each level with icons which will help you to distinguish between beginner, intermediate, and advanced exercises. Eventually, your goal will be to perform the entire series, including all the exercises on the complete Method Workout list, which follows.

Remember the pre-exercises? Before beginning your actual workout, be it level 1 or 2, I suggest performing the pre-exercises for a few weeks at least. They will serve as a thorough preparation to reinforce the principles of the Method Workout each time you do them. After a few weeks, you may no longer feel the need for the pre-exercises and can simply move directly to your workout level.

Progress from one level to the next (according to the plan detailed in chapter 4) by adding exercises, one or two at a time, from the next higher level to your own. Never omit an exercise as you advance but, rather, continually refine and build upon each one of them until all are incorporated into the original and complete Method Workout. Don't be in a hurry. It takes time to develop strength and endurance, to learn how to breathe and build your core. It takes time to learn a new language, and the Method *is* a new language, a reeducation of your muscles as well as your body and mind. Have patience as you work through each movement, each exercise, each series. Being in the moment offers rich rewards, so get ready.

All you have to do is direct your energy toward the desired results and your entire body will be transformed.

THE
COMPLETE
METHOD
WORKOUT

ᛣ	Kapalabhati Breathing	90
ᛣ	Roll-Down	92
ᛣ	Pull-Down	94
ᛣ	Head and Body Roll	96
ᛣ	The Hundred	98
ᛣ	Pre-Roll-Up	100
ᛣ	Roll-Up	102
ᛣ	Leg Circles	104
ᛣ	Rolling Like a Ball	106
ᛣ	Single-Leg Pull	108
ᛣ ᛣ	Double-Leg Stretch	110
ᛣ ᛣ	Scissors	112
ᛣ ᛣ	Double-Leg Lower Lift	114
ᛣ ᛣ	Crisscross	116
ᛣ ᛣ	Pelvic Lift with Leg Extension	118
ᛣ	Spine Stretch Forward	120
ᛣ	Open-Leg Rocker	122
ᛣ ᛣ	Corkscrew	126
ᛣ ᛣ	Saw	128
ᛣ	Pillow	130
ᛣ	Cat-Cow Combination	132
ᛣ	Active Moving Cat	134
ᛣ ᛣ	Active Cat with Yoga Press	136
ᛣ	Cobra	138
ᛣ	Single-Leg Kick	140
ᛣ ᛣ	Double-Leg Kick	142
ᛣ	Child's Pose	144
ᛣ	Flat Yoga Press	146
ᛣ ᛣ	Plank with Battements	148
ᛣ	Down Dog	150

⏣⏣	Down Dog Nose to Knee	152
⏣⏣	Neck Pull	154
⏣⏣⏣	Rollover	156
⏣⏣	Spine Twist	158
⏣	Seated Forward Bend	160
	Side Series	162
⏣	Pendulum	164
⏣	Toss-Up	166
⏣⏣	Bicycle	168
⏣⏣	Inner Thigh Crossover	170
⏣⏣⏣	Ronde de Jambe	172
⏣⏣⏣	Hot Potato	174
⏣⏣⏣	Jackknife	176
	Teaser Series	178
⏣	Single-Bent-Leg Teaser	178
⏣⏣	Classic Teaser	180
⏣⏣	Arms-to-Ears Teaser	182
⏣	Swimming	184
⏣	Seal	186
⏣⏣⏣	Boomerang	188
⏣⏣⏣	Incline Plank	192
⏣	Sun Salutation	194
⏣⏣	Hip Flexor Series with Lunges	200
⏣⏣	Sun Salutation Warrior II	202
	Plié Series	204
⏣	First Position	204
⏣	Second Position	206
⏣	Tendus en Croix	208
⏣⏣	Dégagé	210
⏣⏣	Fondu	212
	Standing Sculpting Series	214
⏣	90-Degree Front Press Forward	214
⏣	Strongman	216
⏣⏣	Side Bend	218
⏣⏣	Chest Expansion	220
⏣⏣	Boxing	222
⏣⏣	Shaving the Head	224
⏣⏣⏣	Hug	226
⏣⏣⏣	Arm Circles	228
	Post-Sculpting Relaxation	230
⏣	Alternate Nostril Breathing	232
⏣	Meditation	234
⏣	Savasana	236

THE COMPLETE METHOD WORKOUT

Act as if what you do makes a difference. It does.

—William James

KAPALABHATI BREATHING

Strengthens the heart and increases lung capacity. Clears the mind and warms up the body, preparing it for exercise.

1. *Sit on the floor in a kneeling position or on your knees.*
2. *Inhale and exhale deeply through your nose. In the next breath, inhale through the nose, filling your lungs only about two-thirds full. Immediately exhale with a quick blast through the nose or the mouth, contracting your abdominals sharply. Immediately inhale again and exhale. Repeat 10 times. As your stamina improves, you should be able to work your way up to 29 inhale/exhales or blasts.*
3. *On your tenth exhalation, continue exhaling until the lungs are empty, and then inhale as deeply as you can, sweeping your arms up overhead and hooking your thumbs together as you apply the three locks: anal, abdominal, and throat (see pages 34–35)*
4. *Hold the breath as long as you comfortably can. When you can hold the breath no longer, lift the chin and, looking straight ahead, exhale and allow the arms to float back down to your sides.*

Now take a few simple ujjayi breaths (see page 38), and after your third or fourth one, begin the second round of kapalabhati.

INSIGHT

When you do your kapalabhati, the important thing to focus on is the warm-up aspect of the breathing, to enjoy the idea that simply by breathing deeply and retaining, you are responsible for creating an internal heat (like the combustion engine of a car) that will fuel your entire workout. Kapalabhati is a good way to register your energy level, your focus, and your attention. Think of it as "diving off the board" into the unique, ever changing landscape of yourself.

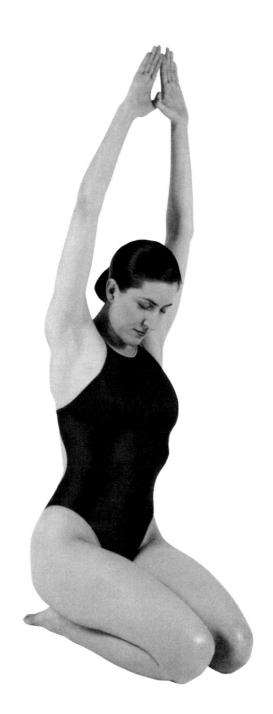

ROLL-DOWN (DANCE AND YOGA)

Opens the backs of the legs and awakens and warms the hamstring connection to the lower back; releases tension in the back, neck, and shoulders through complete spinal articulation.

1. *Stand tall with your feet parallel, arms hanging naturally down by the sides of the body. Inhale deeply and exhale slowly. Feel the crown of the head spiraling up to the ceiling in the same way a barber shop pole's colors swirl in an upward spiral.*

2. *Maintaining the height you have established, draw the navel to the spine, inhale once again, and as you exhale, drop the chin to the chest and start to allow the body to roll forward down toward the floor, one vertebra at a time. (The arms should be heavy, the head and neck and shoulders relaxed; simply allow gravity to do its work.)*

3. *Roll down as far as you are able. Soften the knees and check again that your upper body is free of tension and your breathing is natural.*

4. *Shake your head gently as if saying no. Keep the knees completely bent so that the chest is resting on the thighs, cross your arms at the elbows in front of the legs so your arms become one unit, and continue to hang your head and upper body down.*

5. *Gently and slowly straighten your legs while attempting to maintain the connection of your chest to your thighs.*

6. *Once your legs have reached full extension (you'll feel a keen awareness of your hamstrings), release the arms down to the floor, and inhale here. Exhale as you start to roll up to the starting position, bone by bone through the spine, finally lifting the head, chin, and eyes, until you are standing taller than when you first began.*

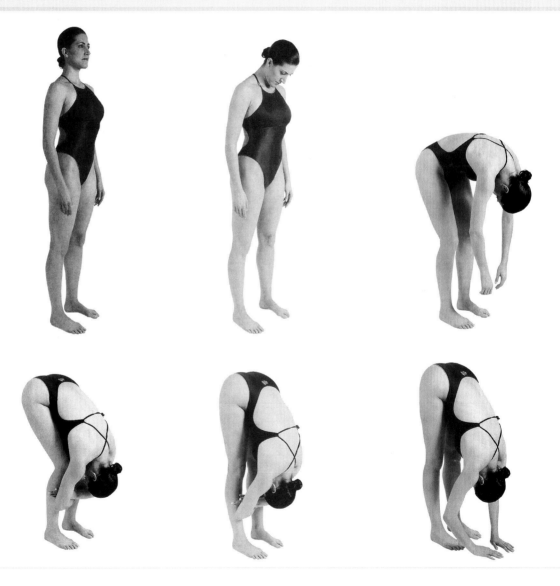

The goal of this exercise is to warm up the spine, free the upper body of any anticipatory tension, and activate the connection between the abdominals and the articulation of the spine . Consider this the first stretch of the day in the legs and the body as a whole. Repeat 2 more times. When I do roll-downs, I think of surrendering to gravity from the very moment I drop my chin to my chest. Pay attention to your back, the degree of flexibility in your hamstrings, your balance, and the use of your breath in tandem with spinal articulation.

PULL-DOWN
(DANCE)

Warms up the quadriceps and hamstring insertions into the gluteals, stretches and strengthens the muscles of the legs and the back, enhances coordination and balance.

1. *After your last roll-down, while standing tall, reach your arms up alongside your ears and try to touch the ceiling without changing the placement of your shoulders. Look up toward the ceiling, lifting your head with support—don't allow it to drop too far back.*

2. *Grasp the air in your fists as you pull down, as if you were pulling a sheet (shoulder width) down from a high shelf, and as you pull down with your elbows, at the same time bend your knees and arch your back as if you were about to sit into a chair.*

3. *Just before you sit, straighten your legs and assume a flat-back position. Place the arms by your sides, parallel to your back, with the fingertips stretching far behind you. Eyes should be looking directly down at the floor. Pull the navel to the spine.*

4. *Inhale. As you exhale, curl the tailbone underneath you so the body assumes a C shape, head also dropped down slightly to complete the C shape through the spine.*

5. *At your sides, curve the arms under, bending at the elbows, as though scooping the folded sheet up into your forearms. Lift the arms up slightly higher and straighten, then drop them straight by your sides, mimicking the movement progression of the back, which is now almost fully erect, and roll the shoulders to prepare for the next "pulling of the sheet down from the shelf" and arching of the back. Repeat the Pull-Down 4 times.*

INSIGHT

Now you'll feel that you are really starting to move and wake up every part of your body, and you'll probably want to listen to some great music, a rich Afro-Celt mix or Stevie Wonder or the Beatles. You pick, but make it something upbeat and inspiring, because now you are dancing, slowly and thoroughly articulating through several different planes of movement and in a few different ranges of motion, building your foundation, enjoying your body.

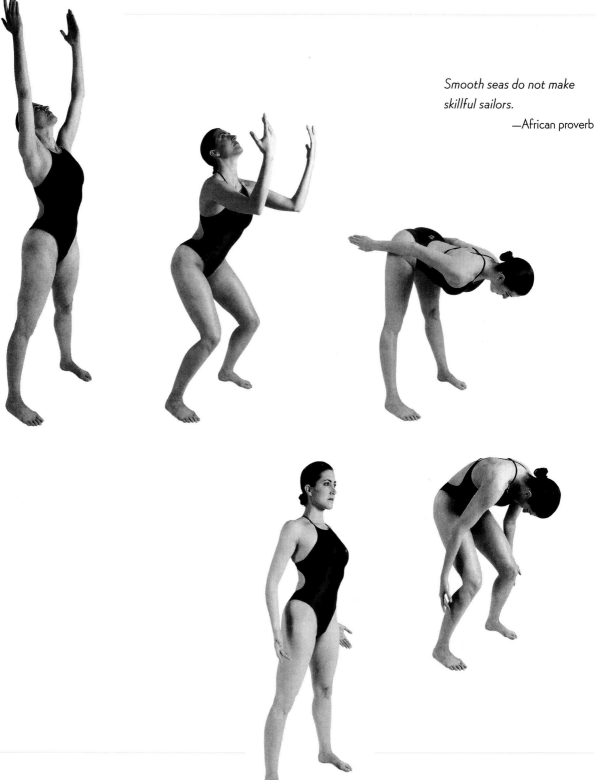

Smooth seas do not make skillful sailors.

—African proverb

HEAD AND BODY ROLL (DANCE)

Warms up the muscles of the head, neck, and shoulders and the upper and lower back, and continues to strengthen the muscles of your legs and fine-tune your balance and coordination.

1. *Stand tall with feet hip width apart, shoulders down and back. Inhale, and as you exhale, drop your right ear toward your right shoulder.*
2. *Slowly circle your head forward and down, then upward toward your left shoulder, and return to your starting position. Repeat the head roll 4 times to the right and then reverse and roll 4 times to the left.*
3. *Start your next circle by involving more of the upper body. Bend the knees so that they are over the toes, and bend your upper torso to the right side of your body. Contract forward slightly as you circle to the left. Arch back again, supporting the head, neck, and now the upper back with the abdominals. Repeat the body rolls 4 times to the right and then switch to the left to circle 4 more times.*

INSIGHT

Work with gravity and allow the weight of your head and upper torso to fall naturally toward the floor. Feel as though you were moving underwater during the entire exercise—this will help you to move smoothly and gracefully.

After the head and body rolls, standing tall, cross your arms in front of your chest and reach the crown of the head toward the ceiling. Pulling the navel to the spine, lower your body to the mat with control, sit down and roll down onto your spine to begin the Hundred. All the following exercises flow like a choreographed dance—one exercise moving smoothly into the next—and your transitions are just as important as the exercises themselves; they are effective moments in which you can condition and tone your abdominals and back while lengthening and strengthening your arms and legs.

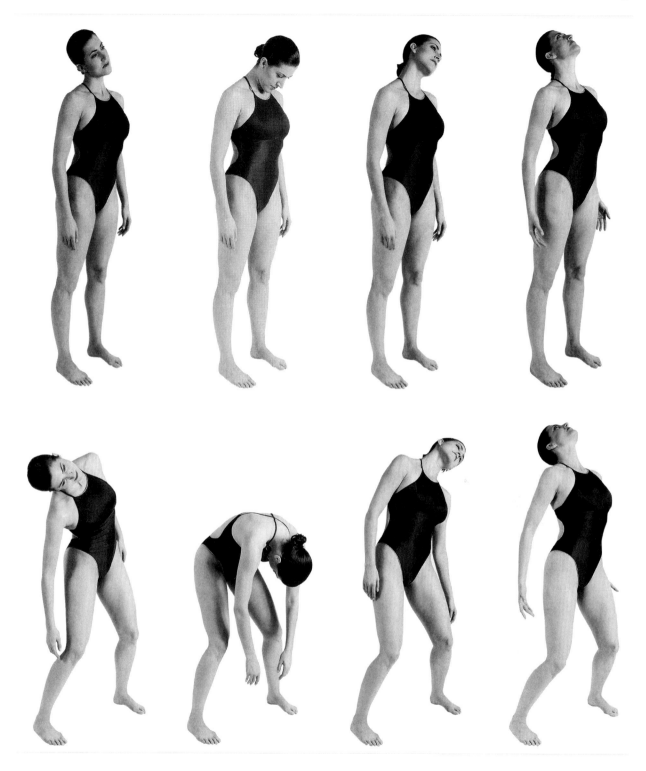

HEAD AND BODY ROLL

THE HUNDRED (PILATES)

The Hundred is the first exercise performed in the Pilates sequence, used to get the blood pumping and the lungs working. It also strengthens the abdominals (targets the rectus abdominus and transversus abdominus) and the muscles in the arms and shoulders.

1. *Lying on your back, draw your knees to your torso, arms extended by your sides. With your navel to your spine, inhale through the nose, and as you exhale, lift the chin to the chest, eyes focused on the abdominals, arms lifted about 3 inches off the floor.*

2. *Extend the legs toward the ceiling at your point of control, where the back remains flat and your abdominals are engaged in supporting your legs. This should be a 75- to 90-degree angle when you begin. (This exercise can be modified to suit you, if you are a beginner or are coming back from an injury, by bending the knees slightly or by keeping them fully bent, as in the first photo.) Keep your heels together and toes flared slightly apart, engaging the inner thigh connection.*

3. *Keep your arms rigid and pump the arms vigorously in tandem with your breathing. The arms are extended directly alongside the body out from the hips with the fingertips reaching toward the opposite wall. Breathe and pump the arms rather quietly, lifting them up to 5 inches and coming immediately back down to their lowest point at your sides to 2 inches off the floor each time you pump. Breathe in for 5 counts and out for 5. Repeat until you have counted 100 inhale/exhales, and continue to maintain the position of the body, with legs up at a right angle and eyes focused on the navel.*

Note: *As you get stronger, lower your legs more toward the floor. If your neck should grow tired when you are starting out, feel free to lower your head to the floor and simply do a set of 50 pumps as opposed to 100.*

INSIGHT

As you are performing the Hundred, imagine that you are trying to bring your forehead toward your thighs. The legs float effortlessly above the action, growing longer as you pump the arms, creating heat in the body and core strength.

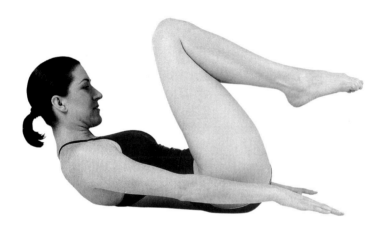

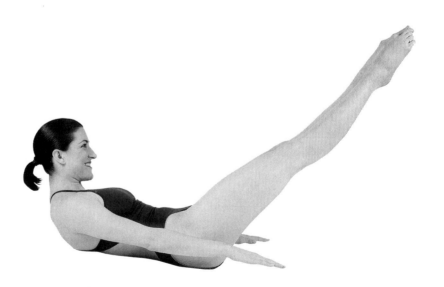

PRE-ROLL-UP (PILATES)

Strengthens the abdominals (rectus abdominus and transversus abdominus) and the muscles of the back. Enhances spinal articulation and massages the back, increasing circulation to the lower back in particular.

1. *Lie on your back, arms extended by your sides, knees bent and together, feet pressing firmly into the floor. Pull the navel to the spine as you extend your arms over your head to your ears. Hands should be 3 inches above the floor.*
2. *Inhale, and exhale as you raise your fingertips toward the ceiling. Using your core muscles, peel your body off the floor as high as you can go, one vertebra at a time, reaching your fingertips forward toward the wall in front of you.*
3. *Inhale at your highest point, with fingertips fully extending toward the wall in front of you, and exhale as you curl your body down, placing one vertebra on the floor at a time until the body has returned to its starting position. Repeat this exercise 5 to 7 times.*

Note: *When you first start out with this exercise you may not be able to lift all the way off the floor to a tall sitting position, but have patience, as your strength increases, so will your level of ability and execution of this and every other exercise. For a modification, you may place your hands behind your knees to assist in peeling the body off the floor.*

INSIGHT

As you do the Pre-Roll-Up, feel as though someone were pulling your fingertips toward the wall in front of you in the first portion of the exercise and helping you to resist the pull of gravity on the way down as you curl back onto the floor.

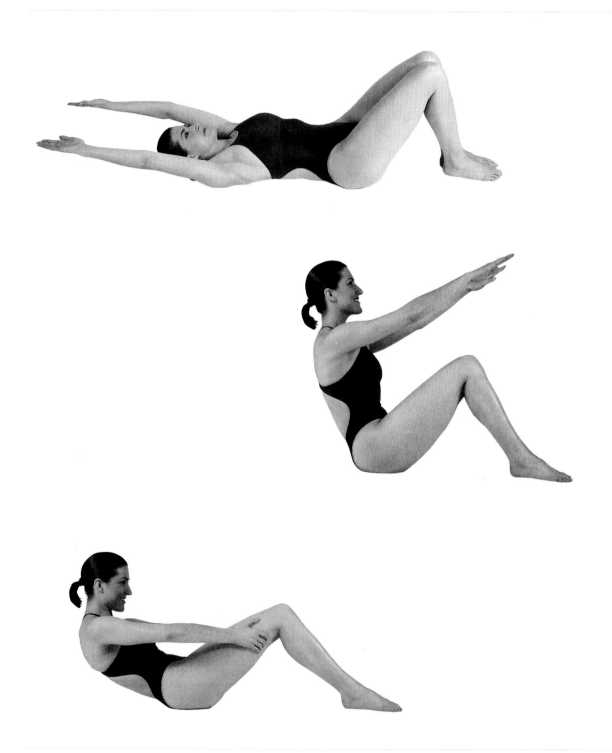

ROLL-UP
(PILATES)

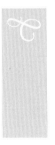

Strengthens the abdominals (rectus abdominus and transversus abdominus) and stretches the hamstrings, calf muscles, and lower back, massaging the spine and enhancing spinal articulation and overall flexibility.

1. *Lie flat on your back, arms extended to the ears overhead, 3 inches above the floor, legs long, with feet squeezing together and flexed.*
2. *Pull the navel to the spine so the small of your back is pressing almost completely against the floor. Inhale, reaching the arms to their full extension, and exhale as you lift your fingertips toward the ceiling and then toward the toes, curling your body off the mat one vertebra at a time.*
3. *Maintaining the curve in your spine, reach as close to your feet as possible. Keep the height of the hands just above the feet.*
4. *With legs pressing down into the floor, quadriceps engaged, inhale, and exhale as you slowly curl back to the floor (push your heels away from you) to assume the initial starting position. Repeat this exercise 5 to 7 times.*

INSIGHT

The key word is *peel*. Make sure you feel as though you were literally peeling your body off the mat bone by bone the way you peel a fruit roll-up away from its wrapper as you curl up and reach the fingertips toward the toes. This can be a frustrating exercise (on a scale of 1 to 10, a definite 9.5). If you experience difficulty with it, you may use your hands to assist you. Come up as high off the floor with your upper body as possible, and then when you reach the point where you feel stuck, use your hands by placing them under your knees as you bend them slightly, and help yourself up the rest of the way; eventually you will rely entirely on the newly developed strength of your abdominals.

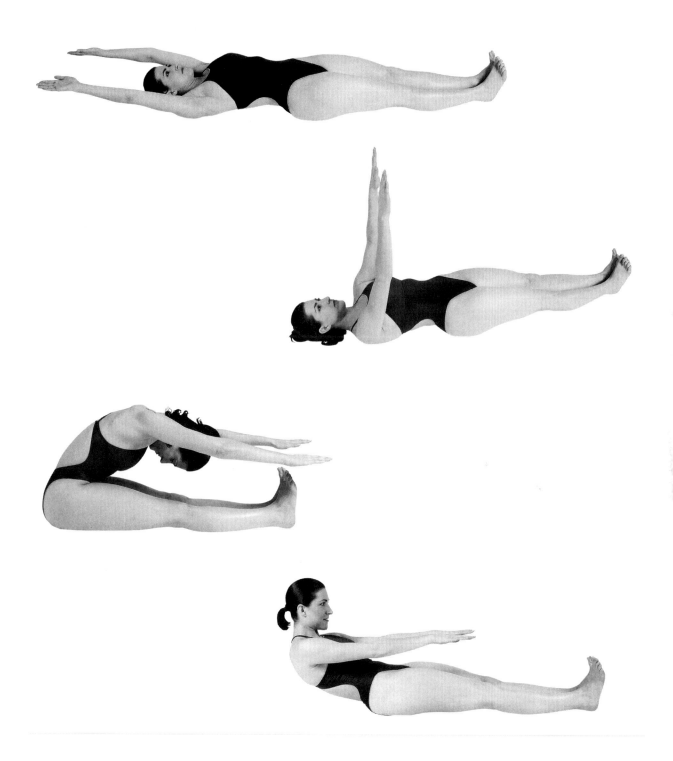

LEG CIRCLES (PILATES)

Strengthens the quadriceps and stretches the hamstrings, toning the muscles of the inner thigh, upper leg (rotator muscles), hip, and buttocks. Strengthens the abdominals and muscles of the lower back through stabilization of the pelvis and core. It requires that you really focus on keeping your navel to the spine as you proceed with the legs. Challenging!

1. *Lie on your back, hands at your sides. Hug your right knee to the chest and extend your right leg up toward the ceiling (form a right angle with the leg) as you concentrate on pulling the navel to the spine.*

2. *Stretch the left leg long on the floor, extending it exactly down the center of the body. Establish symmetry and balance in the body by making sure that your hips are square. Take in a deep breath as you engage the muscles in the front of the thigh (the quadriceps) of your right leg. Press the backs of the arms against the floor and reach your fingertips down toward your feet.*

3. *Circle the leg above, coming toward the body in a counterclockwise motion, a small, controlled circle, as though you were stirring a pot upside down. Make sure that you truly cross the leg over the left side of the body before taking it back up to center. Repeat this 5 to 10 times, and as you circle the leg across, down, and around in a small circle, exhale, and inhale on the way up as you are preparing to circle again. As you get stronger you should aim to make larger circles with the leg, as long as the opposite hip remains anchored as you circle. After you have completed the last circle, reverse the motion, this time going clockwise 5 to 10 times.*

4. *Once completing both directions, pull the right leg as close to your body as possible, trying to keep it straight, and bring your nose as close to your knee as possible. As you stretch here, take deep, smooth breaths in and out through the nose and make sure that your left leg continues to reach right down the center of the body, stretched as long as possible and anchoring your alignment. Navel to the spine, bring your torso only as high up toward the leg as you are able without experiencing discomfort.*

5. *Once you have finished stretching, hug your right knee to your chest, then lower your head and upper body back to the floor. Repeat the entire series on your left leg. Repeat the circles 5 to 10 times in each direction for each leg, and do the series only one time for each side.*

INSIGHT

When you do the leg circles, imagine that you are stirring a pot of soup upside down, a pot of thick pea soup, so that when you move, even though you are moving in a rather speedy, punctuated way, you move with control and really cross the leg over the opposite side of the body before circling the leg down through center, up and around again. You really have to take your spoon (your leg) and stir every side of the pot, most especially the opposite side, before you start your next circle.

Note: *As you become more advanced, you will move directly from the Roll-Up into the right side of the Leg Circles by lifting your leg straight up from the floor, so that the entire series becomes more of a dance, imitating the actual dance sections of the workout.*

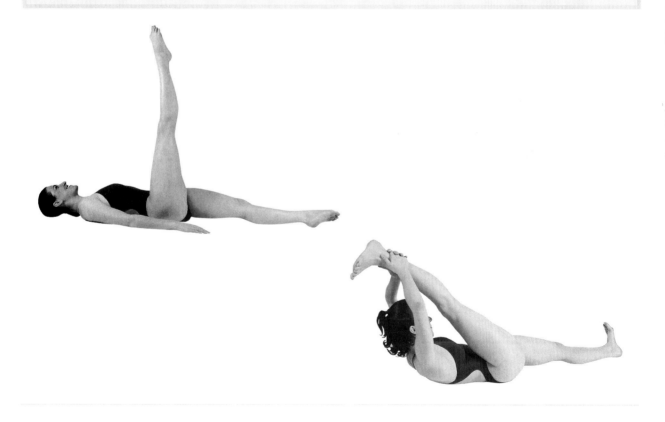

ROLLING LIKE A BALL (PILATES)

Builds abdominal strength (upper rectus), works on coordination and balance, and massages the spine, bringing enhanced circulation to the entire length of the spine and neck.

1. *After you have completed Leg Circles, draw both knees in to your chest (or do the Pre-Roll-Up as a transition to Rolling Like a Ball). As a beginner, you will do a Pre-Roll-Up as a transition to go from lying on your back to sitting up preparing for Rolling Like a Ball. Once you reach the intermediate level, you will be able to "rock up" from the floor and maintain a balance, which is really how Rolling Like a Ball begins.*

2. *Sit up, curl your tailbone underneath you while holding on to your thighs. Once you have found a balancing point (right behind the coccyx—the tailbone), place your hands right on top of your lower shins, above the ankles. Draw your heels toward your buttocks as tightly as possible while establishing a soft point in your feet, toes pointing down toward the floor.*

3. *Make sure that your knees are in line with your shoulders, then lower your head so that it is just between your knees and you are looking at your belly button.*

4. *Relax the shoulders as you inhale and then, exhaling, pull the navel to the spine and the heels toward the buttocks, where they will remain for the duration of the exercise.*

5. *Inhale as you rock the body back in this ball shape, taking care not to rock back too far onto the cervical vertebrae (the neck), and in fact do not touch your head to the mat behind you. Make sure that your heels do not come away from your buttocks and that your abdominals are engaged.*

6. *Exhale as you rock up to the starting position. Hold the minibalance for 3 counts and then repeat the rolling and rocking sequence 5 to 7 times. This exercise is a wonderful spinal massage and an abdominal toning exercise combined.*

INSIGHT

Decide before you begin that you will not allow your heels to separate from your seat, and truly imagine that you are a ball, the tiniest, most compact shape you can conjure in your mind, and when you roll up for the balance, don't get nervous about having to balance in advance, just use the breath to assist you, and relax. Keeping your eyes focused on your navel will help you tremendously.

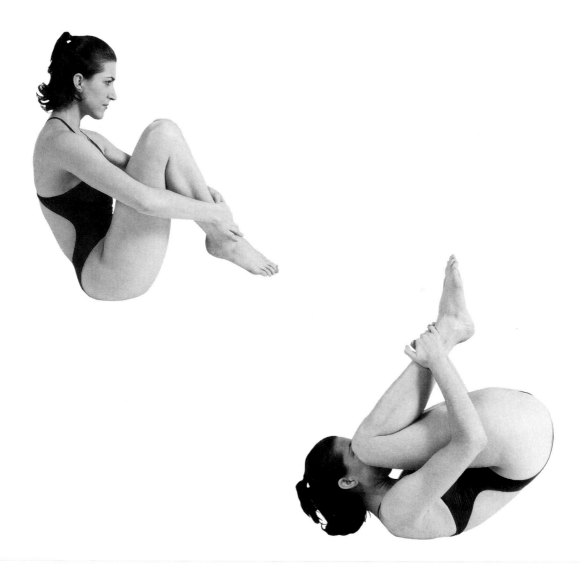

SINGLE-LEG PULL
(PILATES)

Strengthens the abdominals (rectus abdominus and transversus abdominus), enhances coordination, strengthens and lengthens the muscles of the legs and hips.

1. *From Rolling Like a Ball, a smooth transition leads you into Single-Leg Pull. Extend your left leg out in front of the body, reaching it approximately 4 inches off the floor, directly down the midline of the body as you roll down onto your back with control, drawing the right knee in to the chest. This exercise is a bit of a brain teaser and will definitely sharpen your coordination skills.*

2. *Lie on your back. Place your right hand on your right ankle to maintain the leg in proper hip-to-knee alignment and your left hand on your right knee.*

3. *Inhale and double pulse (tug) the bent right leg in toward the face, a pull-pull motion so that you are simultaneously stretching the left leg as far away from the body as possible, creating length in the entire left side of the body.*

4. *As you exhale, switch sides and change your hand positions accordingly: left hand to left ankle, right hand to left knee, and stretch the right leg as far away from the body as you can while drawing the left knee to the nose.*

5. *The eyes are fixed on the navel, and as with all of the Pilates core exercises, the torso is a fixed entity and does not move at all during the exercises. The torso is an anchor for the limbs, creating strength in the abdominal core while the arms and legs move freely, stretching and strengthening through space. You will be tempted to move the head toward the knee in order to achieve the "proper position," but resist the temptation and keep the head still during the exercise. Work harder and more efficiently and draw the knee to the face, which means you will be working your abdominals more effectively.*

6. *Remember to inhale as you pull right and exhale as you pull left, and as you progress to the higher levels, you will breathe as follows: inhale, inhale (small inhale, bigger inhale) on the right and exhale, exhale on the*

left, thereby increasing the breathing challenge and hence increasing
lung capacity.
Repeat this exercise 5 to 7 times.

INSIGHT

Imagine that your torso is cemented to the floor and that when you pull your knee in toward your chest and stretch the opposite leg out, only your legs move. Think of bringing your knee to your nose and of touching the big toe of the outstretched leg to the opposite wall. This way you will create maximum length in your legs and abdominals.

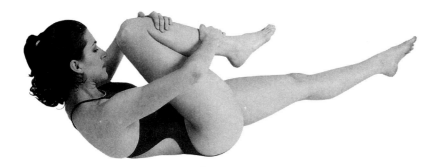

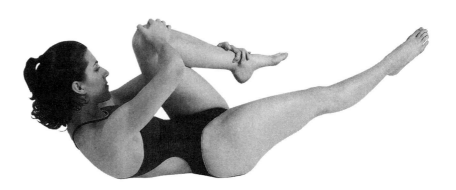

DOUBLE-LEG STRETCH (PILATES)

Strengthens the muscles of the abdominal wall, with an emphasis on the rectus abdominus and transversus abdominus and the muscles of the lower back. Encourages perseverance and determination.

1. *Lie on your back. Draw your knees to your chest and take hold of your ankles. Raise the head up so the forehead is as close to the knees as possible and the shoulder blades are cresting off the floor. Relax your shoulders and pull the navel toward the spine.*

2. *As you inhale, apply even more effort to pulling the navel to the spine and extend the arms straight back behind your head, in line with your ears. Straighten your legs and lift them toward the ceiling. Your head pulls toward your chest, your lower back remains against the floor.*

3. *Hold this position, extending the limbs away from each other in opposition, pointing your toes and reaching your fingertips to their full extension. The eyes remain fixed on the navel and the shoulders are relaxed.*

4. *As you exhale, sweep the arms across the body down by your side and hug the knees to the chest.*
   Repeat 5 to 7 times.

INSIGHT

Try to touch the wall behind you with your fingertips and the wall in front of you with your toes so that you maximize your full-body stretch through opposition. As you extend your legs away from you, imagine you have a large pile of books on your midsection that anchors your torso to the floor. The most important thing to remember is to keep your head lifted in exactly the same place as when you have the knees bent and tucked in toward the upper body. Don't change a thing in your upper-body placement and you will get stronger each time you do this exercise.

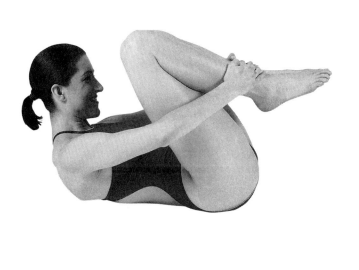

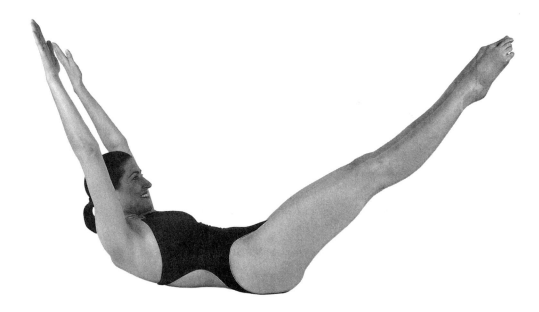

DOUBLE-LEG STRETCH   III

SCISSORS
(PILATES)

Lengthens the hamstrings, strengthens the abdominals, and challenges the body to maintain control at a faster tempo.

1. *Lie on your back; draw both knees to your chest, forehead to the knees.*
2. *Extend the left leg and lower it until it's about 3 inches off the floor. At the same time, extend the right leg toward the ceiling while holding on to the ankle or calf with both hands.*
3. *Keep your chin close to your chest and your eyes are focused on the navel. Make sure that your arms are extended completely and that you are not holding excess tension in your upper neck and shoulders. Inhale as you double-pulse (pull-pull) the right leg toward the body, attempting to keep both legs as straight as possible, then switch legs as you exhale.*
4. *Like the Single-Leg Pull, you can increase the challenge by switching the breath to an inhale-inhale, exhale-exhale as you pull the legs toward your body.*
   Repeat 5 to 7 sets.

Note: *When you first begin this exercise, you may not be able to straighten your legs entirely, but with practice and perseverance, you will certainly increase the flexibility not only in your hamstrings but in your body as a whole.*

INSIGHT

Make sure your arms are outstretched, grasping either the ankle or the area behind the knee, and that your shoulders are not riding up near your ears. This is a golden opportunity to practice the two important muscle pairings to maximize your efforts: the latissimus-trapezius and the quadriceps-hamstrings (see pages 78 and 80). In order to keep the shoulders down and relaxed, engage your latissimus dorsi (the muscle under your armpits on your back attaching to the bottom of the shoulder blade) and then, as you know, you will be able to engage the abdominals more efficiently. Also, engage your quadriceps each time you bring your leg up toward the ceiling, and you will find that your range of motion in the hamstring increases.

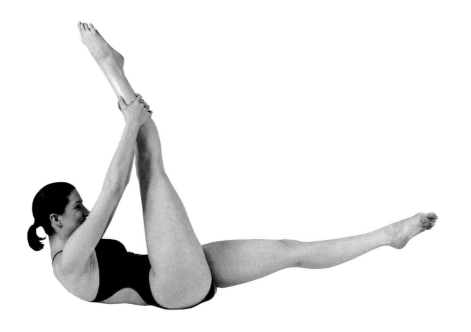

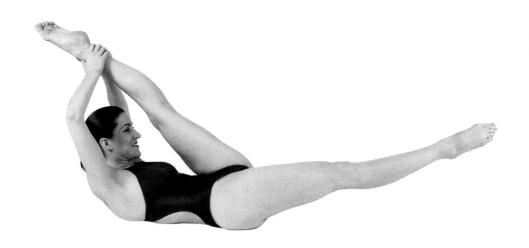

DOUBLE-LEG LOWER LIFT (PILATES)

Another super abdominal strengthener for pyramidalis and rectus abdominus, one that is extremely challenging and empowering. Moves at a slightly faster, punctuated tempo.

1. *Lie on your back and bring your hands behind your head and neck, interlacing your fingers so they form a support for your head.*
2. *Draw your knees to your chest and try to bring your forehead as close to your knees as possible. Inhale, and as you exhale, extend the legs straight up to the ceiling, making sure your navel is pulling in toward the spine, your heels are together, and your toes are apart and pointed.*
3. *Feel the inner thighs squeezing together as you inhale again and maintain the upper torso, keeping the chin as close to the chest as possible. Make sure that the elbows are wide, and the shoulders should be relaxed.*
4. *Inhale again, and as you exhale, lower the legs straight down in front of the body, just to that place where the abdominals connect to the feeling of challenge and the back remains supported and flat against the floor— your point of control. The exercise is dynamic and should be performed with a rather fast, stacato rhythm, lowering the legs slowly then bringing them back up to the starting position in one swift motion.*
5. *Inhale as you again extend the legs back to the starting point, and lower, lower, lower the legs on the exhale. Inhale again and bring the legs up and lower them again on the count of 3.*
   Repeat 5 to 7 times.

INSIGHT

Keep your forehead as close to your thighs as possible. Make sure that you don't lift the legs past a right angle when raising them back up to the ceiling to the starting position. You should lower your legs rather slowly, envisioning a large strap across your middle anchoring your torso to the floor (the way Barbie dolls are held in place on their cardboard backings before you take them out of the package), but then bring the legs back up with a sharp, brisk, controlled tempo and movement, "putting the brakes on" with your abdominals.

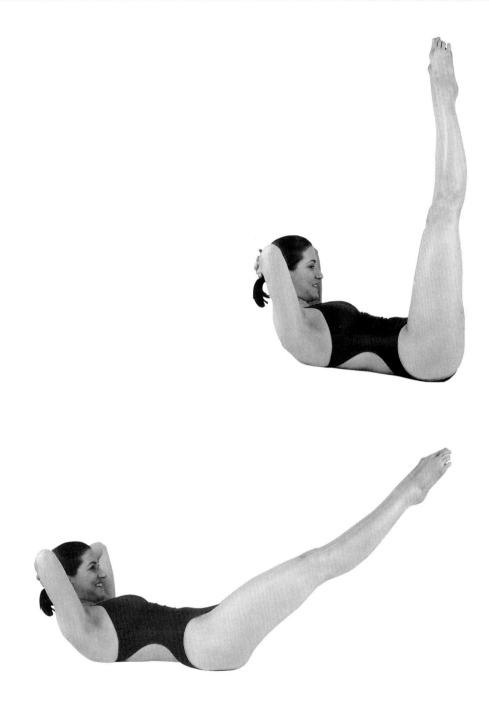

CRISSCROSS (PILATES)

Strengthens the internal and external obliques, rectus abdominus, pyramidalis—a complete abdominal toner. Because of the twisting nature of the exercise, it massages the internal organs. Lengthens the muscles of the legs and hips. Medium tempo.

1. *Lie on your back and draw both knees to the chest. Place your hands behind the head at the base of the neck with fingers interlaced. Bring your forehead as close to the knees as possible. Inhale, and on the exhale, draw the right knee toward the left elbow as you fully extend the left leg down the midline of the body approximately 4 inches off the ground.*

2. *Open your right elbow behind you and look beyond the open elbow as you fully twist the torso; see the wall behind you as you aim to touch the left elbow to the knee. Inhale here, and exhale as you switch to the other side. Throughout the exercise, make sure to keep the torso anchored and as still as possible so as to maximize the use of the abdominals.*
Repeat 5 to 7 sets.

INSIGHT

Here again, imagine that the torso is anchored to the floor with a pile of books. Be careful not to "rock the boat," not to shift the torso side to side as you bring the knee in to meet the elbow or the books will topple. The key to this exercise is to keep the torso perfectly still as you pull the knee in to meet the elbow, not the other way around. Try it both ways and feel the difference. You will find that you have to invest more focus and effort when you pull the knee in toward the body first. Also, don't forget to really see the wall behind you each time you twist.

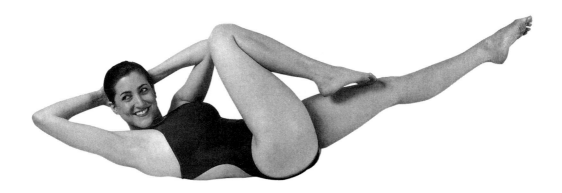

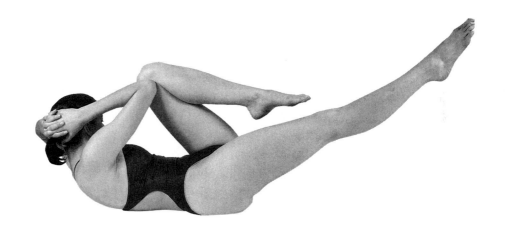

PELVIC LIFT WITH LEG EXTENSION (PILATES AND YOGA)

Strengthens the hamstrings, cultivates symmetry and balance between the two sides of the body. Inspires patience and devotion.

1. *Lie on your back with both knees bent, hip width apart, feet firmly pressing against the floor, arms down at the sides of the body. Inhale, and as you exhale, lift the hips to the ceiling, making sure to pull the navel to the spine and tilt the pelvis slightly upward (tucking) so as to control the arch in the lower back.*

2. *The knees are directly in line with the toes and the arms continue to press against the floor, serving as added leverage for the body. Inhale, and as you exhale, roll down through the spine one vertebra at a time, gently massaging the spine against the floor.*

3. *Inhale again and exhale, pressing the hips up to the ceiling; extend the right leg up to the ceiling, pointing the toes—you should feel as though you are attempting to touch the ceiling with your foot. Press the left foot firmly against the floor and make sure the hips are lifting up to the ceiling evenly so that the hamstring of the left leg is being stretched.*

4. *Inhale, and as you exhale, slowly lower the straight right leg down to 5 inches above the floor as you flex the foot. Inhale, lift the leg back up to starting position, where you'll once again point the foot with control. Repeat this lower and lift 5 times.*

5. *After the last repetition, when the right leg is approximately 4 inches above the floor, bend the right knee and place your foot back on the floor. Roll down through the spine one vertebra at a time. Inhale, and as you exhale, lift the hips to the ceiling once again and repeat the entire series with the left leg.*
   Repeat the full sequence, right and left leg, 2 times.

INSIGHT

As you lift your hips toward the ceiling, imagine that you are being suspended from the ceiling by a harness under your buttocks. Fully engage each leg as you kick it up toward the ceiling and as you lengthen it down with control. You will find that it feels lighter if you stretch it completely.

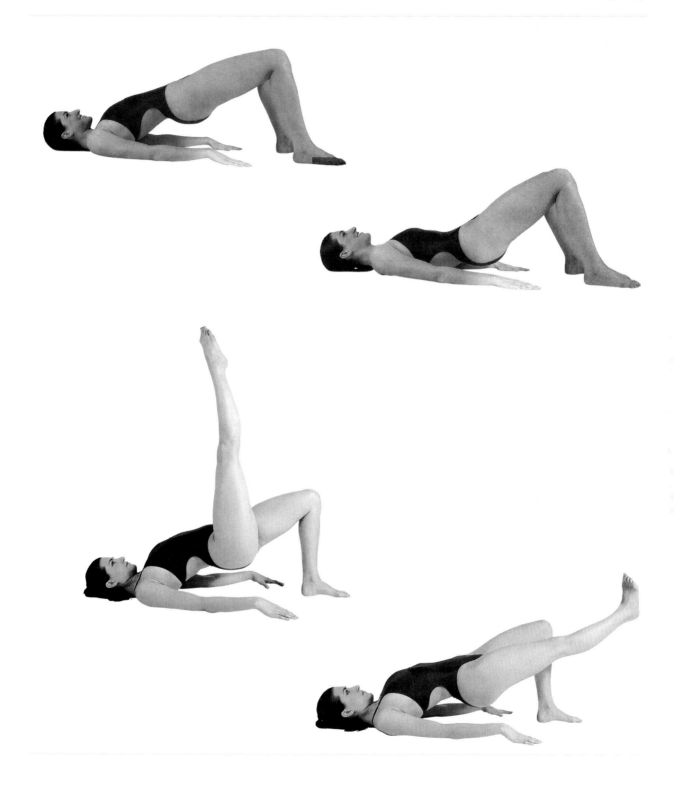

PELVIC LIFT WITH LEG EXTENSION

SPINE STRETCH FORWARD (PILATES)

Stretches the spine and muscles of the neck, shoulders, and back, conditions the abdominals, and stretches the hamstring and hamstring insertion into the lower gluteals lumbar (quadratus lumborum). Creates space between the intervertebral discs of your spine, bringing new oxygen and fresh blood to the area. An excellent exercise for counteracting the effects of computer slump.

1. *Sit tall, with legs straight out in front of you, slightly wider than hip width apart. Roll your shoulders down and back. Flex your feet and lift the crown of your head toward the ceiling, imagining your head is just grazing the ceiling. Engage your abdominals to help lengthen your spine and lift your upper body.*

2. *Extend your arms straight out in front of you at shoulder level; take a deep breath in.*

3. *As you exhale, curl your head down, chin to chest, eyes on your navel, and continue to reach your fingertips straight out in front of you. Feel as though someone were hugging you around your middle and pulling you backward as you fight to reach forward in the opposite direction—all the while scooping the abdominals in away from the arms—creating a C shape.*

4. *Inhale and uncurl through the spine, pulling the abdominals in toward the back as you return to "perfect posture." Feet remain flexed and legs extended throughout the entire exercise. Exhale and drop the chin to the chest and repeat the entire sequence 5 to 7 times.*

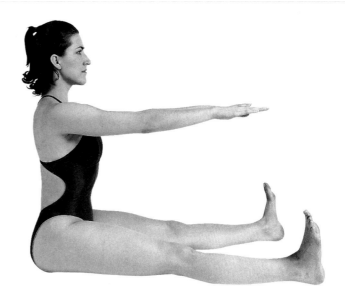

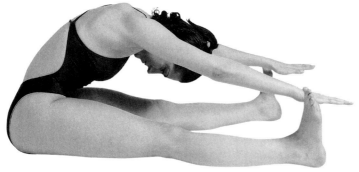

INSIGHT

Try to touch the ceiling with the crown of your head. Lift your spine up out of your hips, as if you had a spring in place of your spine, and stretch the coils of the spring so that there is space between each one. Imagine that you are scooping your belly away from a big beach ball and are not permitted to touch it with your stomach. As you return to the starting position, imagine that you are uncurling your spine against a wall. This exercise helps to establish perfect posture in a seated position and helps you to learn what it feels like to experience length and height in your torso. The next time you sit down in front of your computer, at the breakfast table, or behind the wheel of your car, your body will have developed muscle memory and you will find it easier to assume the proper posture to keep your back feeling tall and pain-free.

OPEN-LEG ROCKER PREP (PILATES)

Strengthens the abdominals, stretches the hamstrings and insertion into the lower lumbar, enhances balance and coordination, and brings increased circulation to the lower back.

Preparation (for Level 1)

1. Begin in the same sitting position as for Spine Stretch Forward, but this time bend your knees and curve your back into a big C shape, scooping the abdominals in and holding on to your legs behind the knees.

2. Shift your weight back so you are balancing just behind your tailbone. Lift your legs up so that your feet are at shoulder height, knees still bent, lower legs parallel to the floor, hands holding lightly behind the knees and eyes focused straight ahead.

3. Inhale and roll backward without touching your head to the mat. Exhale and come back up to balance at the starting position, with the feet returning to shoulder height. Repeat this 5 to 7 times. These rocking motions will bring relief to those of you who suffer from chronic back pain.

4. After rolling back and forth a few times with bent knees, bring your feet back down to your seat (as in Rolling Like a Ball). Hold on to your ankles, extend your legs straight up at an angle in front of you, open them to a V shape, close them back together, and bend them again, returning to the starting position, with the heels toward your seat and feet softly pointed. Repeat this preparation series 3 to 5 times before moving on.

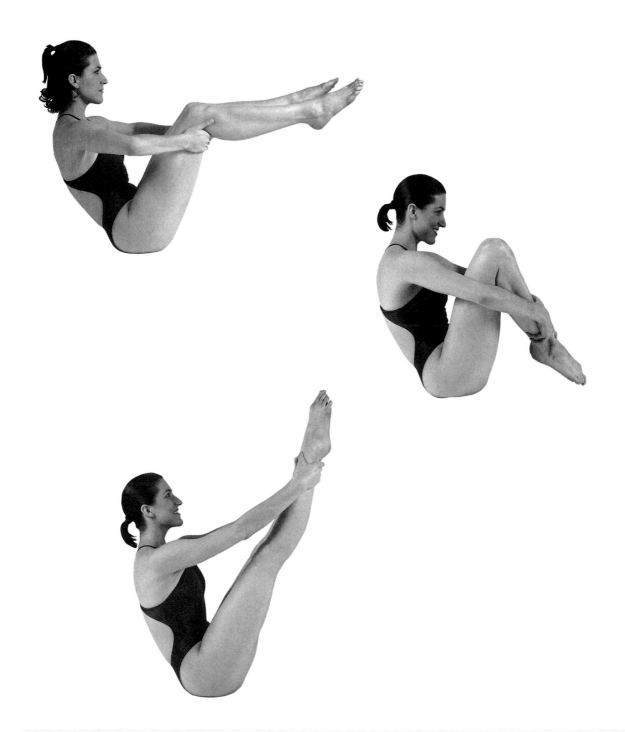

OPEN-LEG ROCKER (PILATES)

1. *Straighten your legs and hold on to your ankles, keeping your legs hip width apart. Breathe in and out with smooth, concentrated breaths as you balance in the upright position with legs extended, feet softly pointed, and abdominals pulled in toward the spine, which should be slightly curved in a tall C position.*

2. *As you inhale, roll back. Do not let go of your legs; you will not derive the same abdominal benefit if you do. Do not allow your head to touch the mat behind you. Exhale and rock with control back up to the starting position. If you're experiencing difficulty returning to the upright balancing position, bend the knees a little.*

   Repeat 5 to 7 times. Have fun with this one.

INSIGHT

After you establish your balance and are preparing to rock backward, have Rolling Like a Ball in mind, as this is the sister exercise. When you rock back, imagine that you are holding a bowl of marbles on your belly. If you rock back too far and allow your head to touch the floor behind you, you will lose your marbles! So make sure that you "put the brakes on" with your abdominals, and do the same as you rock back up. Lift your eyes when you go to rock up; this will assist you in returning to the starting position.

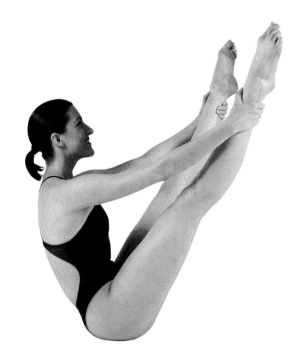

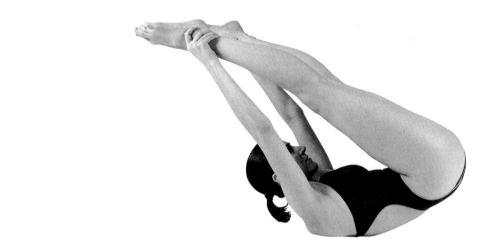

**CORKSCREW
(PILATES)**

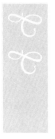

Strengthens the abdominals and lower back, tones the triceps, lengthens the quadriceps, and firms inner thighs.

1. *Lie on your back with your arms down by your side. Draw your knees in to your chest and extend the legs straight up to the ceiling.*
2. *With heels glued together and toes apart and pointed, press the arms against the floor and try to straighten the legs up toward the ceiling as much as possible by engaging the quadriceps (thigh muscles).*
3. *Inhale, and as you exhale, begin to circle the legs by moving them down and toward the right in a counterclockwise motion. Make sure that you concentrate on pulling the navel to the spine as the legs circle in each direction to your point of control.*
4. *Once you've completed the circle and your legs are back in starting position, inhale. As you exhale, circle the legs in the reverse direction. Repeat 4 times in each direction.*

Note: *If you are concerned about your lower back, instead of placing your hands by your sides, you can bring your hands together under your lower back for support.*

INSIGHT

When I do the Corkscrew, I imagine that my lower back is attached to the floor with a large piece of Velcro so that my pelvis stays anchored as I circle my legs. I pretend that I have paintbrushes attached to each foot and that I am painting circles on the ceiling. I concentrate on reaching my legs so far away from my center that my legs become fifteen feet long, and as I circle them down and around, they feel lighter and the movements feel easier.

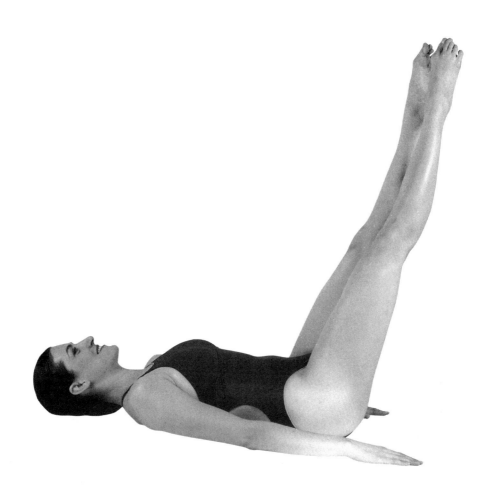

CORKSCREW

SAW
(PILATES)

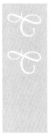

Opens the chest and shoulders. Increases range of motion in the torso, stretching the muscles of the back and waist, and increases flexibility in the hamstrings and lower back. A great breathing exercise for increasing lung capacity, and a powerful antidote for asthma.

1. *Sit tall with legs outstretched, slightly wider than hip width. Extend the arms out to the sides, fingertips reaching as far away from the body as possible. (Make sure that the feet are flexed and that you are pulling the navel to the spine.) Inhale and retain the breath as you twist the body from the waist toward the left leg, bringing the right outstretched arm with you (the left arm is fully stretched behind you).*

2. *As you exhale, "saw" off the baby toe of the left foot with the back of your right hand. Make sure to keep the right leg completely straight and the foot fully flexed. The head is dropped toward the kneecap and the spine is curled forward in the C shape, with the navel to the spine.*

3. *Inhale to return to center. Repeat the sequence on your right side. Repeat 6 sets.*

INSIGHT

Imagine your lower body is sitting in cement when you twist your upper torso against your lower body, so that your hips, legs, and feet are anchored and in alignment with one another as you move through the series. To maximize your movements and increase your flexibility, as you twist and stretch, to the right for instance, flex your left foot (always flex the opposite foot) deeper and press that heel against the floor as much as possible. In this way your opposite side will be well anchored in that cement you are sitting in and you will be free to properly explore your full range of motion on that opposite side.

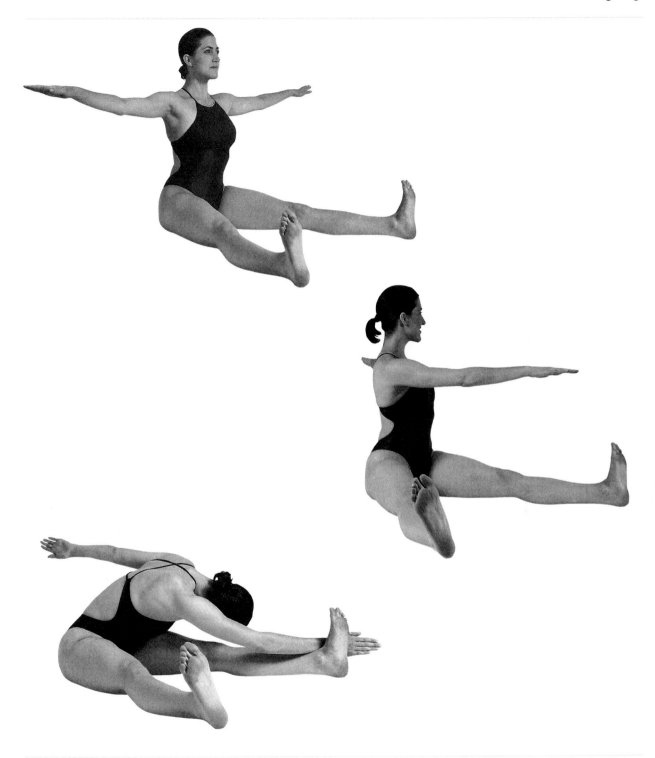

PILLOW
(PILATES)

Isolates and strengthens the abdominals and enhances coordination.

1. *Lying on your stomach, create a pillow by placing your hands together, one on top of the other, and let your head rest on them, either with the nose down to the floor or with the head turned comfortably to one side or the other.*
2. *Inhale and bring your heels together, with legs long and the body relaxed, allowing the full weight of your body to sink into the floor. As you exhale, pull the navel to the spine, defying gravity, imagining that you are pulling your belly away from your belt buckle on a tight pair of jeans.*
3. *Hold the navel to the spine, contracting the abdominals, and inhale while continuing to hold the navel to the spine.*
4. *Relax the abdominals to the floor and note the difference in feeling between the contraction and the release of the abdominals.*
5. *Repeat the action with the breath 3 to 5 times, inhaling and then exhaling as you lift the navel to the spine and hold it there for at least one full breath cycle (meaning inhale and exhale).*

This intense lifting in the abdominal region is the feeling you should have throughout the series whenever you work in a prone position (anytime you do any exercise while lying on your stomach).

INSIGHT

Remember the "pulling your belly away from the tight waistband" scenario from the Essential Elements? This is the sister exercise to that physical moment associated with finding your navel-to-spine connection. This time you will be using the same imagery to engage your abdominals, and this time you will be working against gravity when you do it. This exercise is perhaps the best preparation for all the prone exercises you will do in the workout.

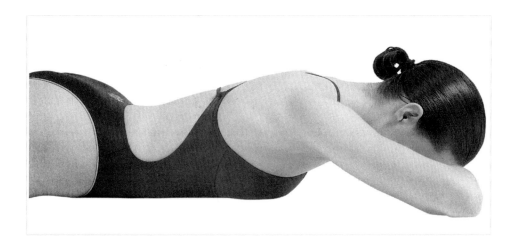

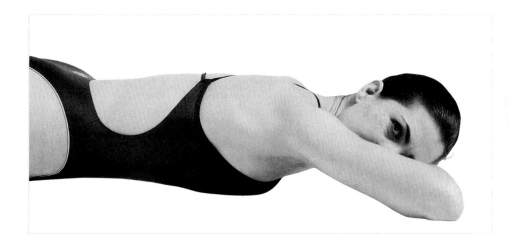

CAT-COW COMBINATION (YOGA)

Opens the spine, releases tension in the muscles of the neck and shoulders, and stretches the palms, the fingers, the feet and toes. This exercise is particularly effective for stretching and opening the spine, the shoulders, and the neck and for counteracting the effects of poor posture.

1. *Assume a dog position, on hands and knees, with your palms spread directly underneath your shoulders. Make sure that your ankles are in line with your knees. The head should be in line with the spine, which is in a flat tabletop position.*

2. *Breathe in, lift the eyes, the chin, and the chest up toward the ceiling while still supporting the neck, and start to arch the back, sticking the tail out behind you, and roll the shoulders back away from the ears. Curl the toes underneath you so you feel a stretch between the toes and the pad of your foot.*

3. *Make sure that your palms are open wide against the floor, and feel that your arms are energized, supporting the upper body maximally.*

4. *As you exhale, curl the spine under, dropping the chin to the chest and tucking the tailbone under the body so that you are in as small a rounded shape as you can assume. The toes curl as well, and the top of the foot simply goes flat against the floor during the curl segment.*
   Repeat this exercise 5 to 7 times.

INSIGHT

Think animal when performing this exercise. Think first movement in the morning after waking up. Think slow and thorough and luxurious. Think gentle and sensual. Even though this exercise comes at a point in the workout after you have already worked quite hard, think of this as a preparation, relaxation, and focusing exercise. Focus on the breath, and the rest will follow.

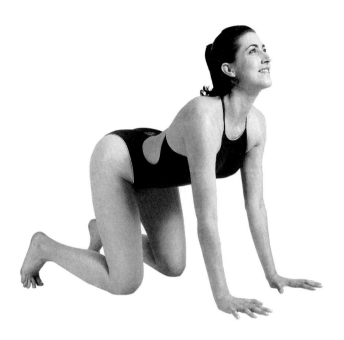

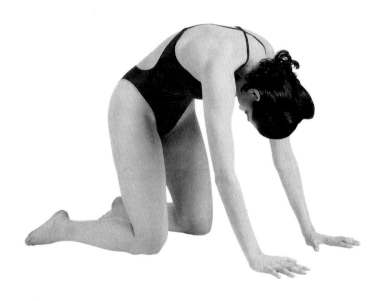

CAT-COW COMBINATION

ACTIVE MOVING CAT (YOGA)

Strengthens and tones the hamstrings and buttocks and muscles of the back (upper and lower) and tones the abdominals.

Let's take the Cat-Cow Combination a step further now.

1. *Start again in the hands-and-knees position. Lift the eyes, chin, and chest up toward the ceiling and lift the right leg straight up behind you as high as you can without overarching the back. Lift the abdominals to support the spine, and press the hands and arms against the floor to support the upper body. Be sure you are pointing the right foot to your fullest extent and that the kneecap is lifted.*

2. *As you exhale, drop the chin to the chest and try to bring the right knee in to touch the forehead. You will feel an extraordinary abdominal pull as you attempt and perform this movement. Repeat the leg lift and tuck 4 times on the right leg and then switch to the left.*

INSIGHT

When you go to extend your leg behind you, imagine that you are underwater and think of having to pull the leg up through the water, so that you move with a certain measure of resistance and control. When you curl your spine under and bring the knee to your nose, imagine that you are a snail or a turtle pulling its head back into its shell.

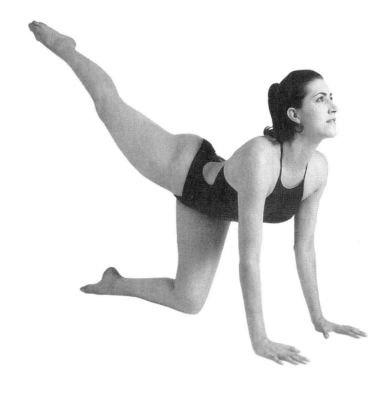

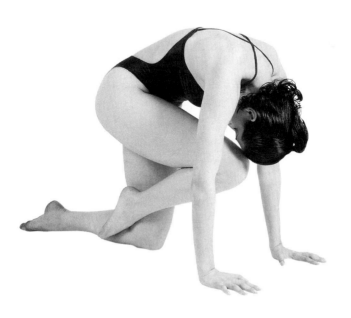

ACTIVE CAT WITH YOGA PRESS (YOGA)

Strengthens the muscles of the upper arms and back, tones the triceps, and conditions the abdominals. An empowering series.

1. *Kneel on your hands and knees; inhale as you lift the eyes, chin, and chest up toward the ceiling; lift the right leg straight up behind you—as high as you can without overarching the back. Engage your abdominals to support the spine and press your hands against the floor to support the upper body. Make sure that you are pointing the right foot to your fullest extent and that the leg muscles are working to their capacity.*

2. *As you exhale, bring the body forward by bending your arms and leveraging with the palms on the floor into a "push-up" or "press" position.*

3. *As you inhale again, you will push the floor away and return to the starting position with the leg fully extended.*

4. *As you exhale, drop the chin to the chest (as you did in the second part of the Cat-Cow Combination) and try to bring the right knee in to touch the forehead. You will feel an extraordinary abdominal pull as you perform this movement. The pulling feeling is the toning of your abdominal wall.*

   Repeat exercise, doing 4 sets on the right and 4 sets on the left.

INSIGHT

Use a waltz rhythm to really get going in this series. It should go something like this: 1-inhale, 2, 3, lift (the leg); 1-exhale, 2, 3, body forward toward the floor; 1-inhale, 2, 3, lift the body up; and 1-exhale, 2, 3, tuck the knee to the nose. Use the floor once again, both resisting it on the way down, as your chest moves forward and down, and then pushing it away from you as you lift the body up. Imagine you are kicking a heavy ball up to the ceiling behind you with your foot. Try to literally touch the ceiling with your foot as you extend it behind you, and aim to bring the chin to the floor as you move forward into the press portion of the series.

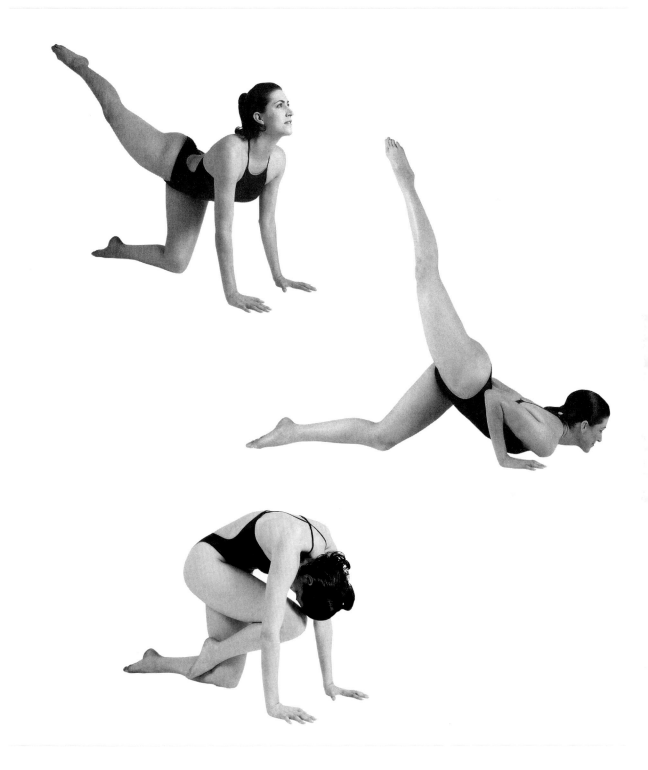

COBRA
(YOGA)

A wonderful back strengthener that will not only help you improve muscle definition in your back (upper and lower), tone and firm your buttocks and the backs of the legs, and prepare you for the more demanding exercises to come but will reinforce correct standing posture.

1. *Lie on your stomach and place your hands directly under your shoulders. Your elbows should be bent, facing up toward the ceiling. Your head should be in line with the spine, forehead gently on the floor. The legs are long and straight behind the body and the heels together.*
2. *Squeeze the buttocks, and as you inhale, lift the eyes, chin, and chest and press the hands against the floor, lifting the upper body so the chest comes off the floor slightly. You should feel the muscles of the back and the abdominals supporting the movement.*
3. *Stay in this position, breathing in and out for 5 breaths, and then relax the body down to starting position.*
Repeat 2 times.

INSIGHT

Imagine that you are a desert creature and you have been asleep for a thousand years. You are finally emerging from your deep sleep, moving with great purpose and control, lifting your body up out of the sand as you defy gravity with the muscles of your upper back and arms. Picture the sphinxes in Egypt, tall, stoic, and proud. This is the Cobra.

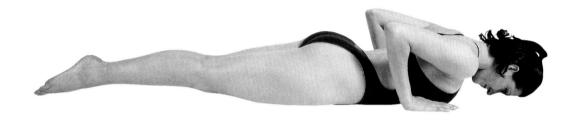

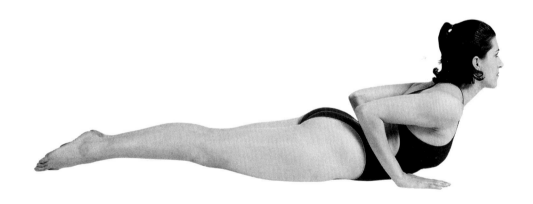

SINGLE-LEG KICK
(PILATES)

Strengthens the back, shapes the buttocks and the backs of the legs, and strengthens the abdominals.

1. *Lie on your stomach, with your upper body propped up on your elbows and fists. Arms should be lined up directly in front of the chest, legs stretched out behind the body, fully extended, with the heels squeezing together.*
2. *Squeeze the buttocks tight and make certain the abdominals are lifting as you bend the left knee and point the toes of the left foot, double-pulsing the foot toward the buttocks. Inhale as you pulse your leg. Exhale as you bring your left leg to the starting position and bend your right leg toward the buttocks, pulsing twice and inhaling, bringing the right heel to the right buttock.*
3. *You will feel the hamstrings, buttocks, and abdominals working as you do this exercise.*
   Perform 5 to 7 sets.

INSIGHT

Instead of thinking about lifting your upper body away from the floor, consider the notion of "pushing the floor away." In addition, when working the legs, stretch them fully against the floor between kicks and think of reaching your big toe along the floor all the way to the wall behind you. When kicking the heel toward the buttocks, imagine there is a bell attached to your backside and each time you hit the bell, you are one step closer to looking like a million bucks in that new swimsuit!

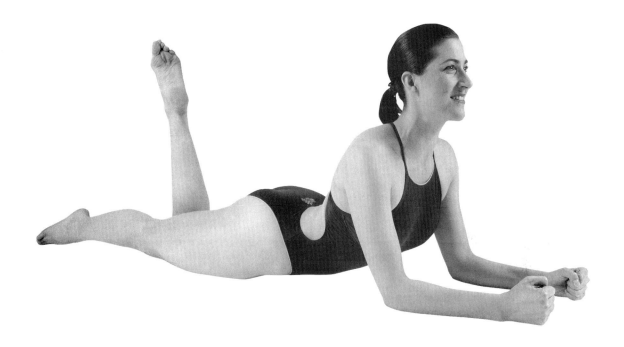

DOUBLE-LEG KICK
(PILATES)

One of the more challenging back exercises, this will help you to both stretch and strengthen your upper back and shoulders (especially useful for all of us who use a computer on a regular basis). Strengthens the back and conditions the hamstrings. Opens the chest and shoulders, stretching all the connective tissue and improving coordination.

1. *Lie on your stomach with your face turned to the right. Your legs are extended behind you with heels together. Clasp your hands behind your back—hold the right index and middle fingers with the left hand. The elbows are bent and touching the floor to the sides of the body.*
2. *Bend the knees, keeping your legs together and toes pointed, as you press the hips against the floor by squeezing the buttocks. Your elbows remain bent and touching the floor this whole time.*
3. *Inhale and pulse (kick) your legs toward the buttocks 3 times. As you exhale, extend your legs and straighten your arms behind your back, lifting the upper body as high off the floor as possible, anchoring the feet to the floor. Hold for a few seconds and relax by coming to rest your left cheek on the floor.*
   Repeat 6 times.

INSIGHT

Pretend you are a mermaid who is frolicking about. In this instance you won't be flipping your tail around aimlessly but will be directing it very specifically, of course. When you bend your knees and bring your feet toward your buttocks three times in rather rapid succession, make sure that the legs and feet come to be glued together (they become the mermaid's tail) and work as one unit. In this way you will also tone your inner thighs—a bonus.

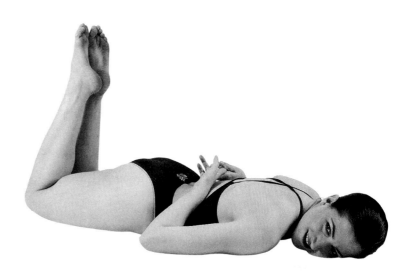

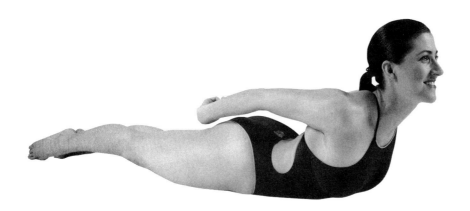

DOUBLE-LEG KICK 143

CHILD'S POSE
(YOGA)

This is a very important rest position that should follow any exercise where you feel the need to relax the spine or be used to take a moment out from your regime when you feel you need a break. Softens the muscles of the entire body, especially those of the lower back, stretching them as well. Relaxes the muscles of the head, neck, and shoulders.

1. *Kneel with your knees slightly apart and sit on your heels.*
2. *With control, bend forward over your knees, bringing your forehead softly to the floor.*
3. *After finding a comfortable position for your head, with the spine rounded forward, buttocks grazing the heels, bring your arms to rest at your sides with your palms facing up toward the ceiling.*
   Rest in child's pose for up to 5 breaths.

INSIGHT

The name used for this asana, Child's Pose, is quite apt, because for me it has always signified something resembling the fetal position. You are not in a completely vulnerable position as you are when you are on your side but facedown, on your knees, paradoxically very much in command of a position that permits surrender. Allow yourself to curl over and release into the floor, giving over entirely to gravity, to rest.

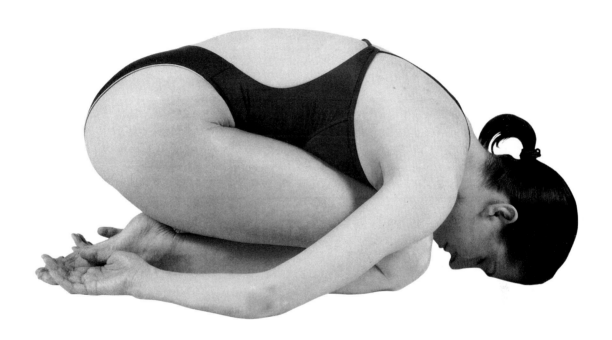

145

FLAT YOGA PRESS (YOGA)

Creates awareness of proper pelvic alignment, strengthens and tones the inner thighs. Strengthens the upper body and arms, tones the triceps, prepares the body for more challenging upper-body strengthening exercises.

Note: Before you begin this exercise, kneel, with the back upright, with the knees squeezing together and the abdominals pulling in toward the spine. Press the arms against the sides of the body, palms against the thighs. Bend the arms at the elbows and squeeze the arms against the body so that there is no space remaining between you and your arms. You will feel the muscles of the upper, inner arm (triceps) engage. Make sure that your spine is tall and straight and your abdominals are lifted. Remember this position, as you will translate it into the actual movement when you go to perform this exercise.

1. *Start on your hands and knees with your back forming a clean tabletop. The head is directly in line with the tailbone, the hands directly under the shoulders, palms spread wide against the floor. Abdominals are lifted up into the spine. Keep the elbows tucked in toward the body and squeeze the knees together.*
2. *Inhale, and with control, bring the body forward, feeling as though someone were pulling you from the crown of the head. The neck is long and the body is in one flat plane (the lower legs and feet should remain anchored to the floor). The elbows remain tucked into the sides of the body as the body shifts forward and the elbows bend farther, bringing the body closer to the floor.*
3. *It is crucial that you bend the elbows only as far as you are able to control the weight of the body as it descends toward the floor. As you get stronger, you will be able to bend the elbows to such a degree that your body will be just a few inches off the floor.*
   As you exhale, pull the body back into the starting position.

INSIGHT

Imagine you have a spring attached to the crown of your head and one attached to your bottom. As you move forward into the press, you move with added control and resistance and are able to maintain a flat-back position instead of allowing the upper body to collapse. As you move backward to return to your starting position, you feel as if you were getting some help, being pulled backward by the spring.

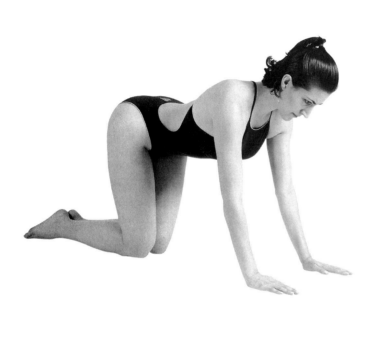

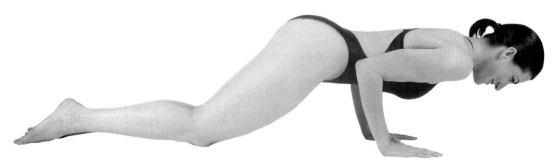

PLANK WITH BATTEMENTS (PILATES)

This exercise, like the Flat Yoga Press, focuses on building upper-body strength but also works on toning and strengthening the body as a whole. It strengthens the back, chest, shoulders, hamstrings, and buttocks.

1. *Begin on your hands and knees with your hands positioned directly underneath your shoulders and your knees exactly hip width apart. Creating a straight line from your head to your rear, extend your right leg directly behind you, curling the toes underneath to support the extended leg.*

2. *Now bring the left leg back in the same manner. Lift your abdominals up into the body to support the spine, and make sure the arms are fully extended. Assume a pelvic alignment with the pubic bone tucked tightly under and the buttocks engaged.*

3. *Inhale and slowly lift the right leg up toward the ceiling, with the foot pointed. Exhale as you flex the foot and lower the leg until it barely touches the floor. Be sure to hold the body firmly in position as you raise and lower the leg. After 5 repetitions, switch to the other leg.*

4. *After completing the 5 repetitions with the left leg, ease the body down onto the hands and knees and curl into Child's Pose (page 144) to rest. Perform 2 sets.*

INSIGHT

One of the most empowering exercises in the workout, the Plank with Battements requires that you maintain the same muscular connections as in the Flat Yoga Press. Keep the buttocks tight so that the pubic bone curls under slightly, which will lengthen the lower back and help you to engage your abdominals more effectively. The tendency is to allow the rear end to lift. Instead, you should tuck your pelvis slightly so that the work of the pose is transferred to your abdominal core.

The word *battement* means to kick and when you perform the "kicking" aspect of this exercise, make sure to control the kick both on the way up and down, so as to sculpt the buttocks more effectively. You should feel as though you have sandbags attached to your ankles so that you move gracefully up and down.

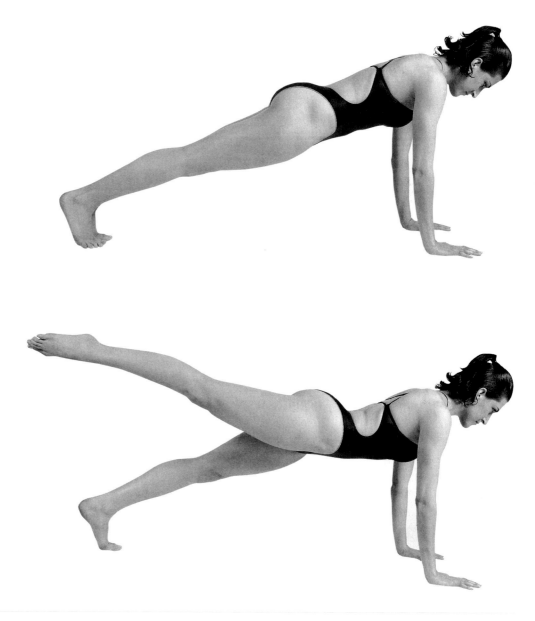

DOWN DOG (YOGA)

Strengthens the muscles of the upper back, chest, and shoulders and tones the quadriceps as it lengthens the muscles of the hamstrings and opens the insertions into the lower back.

1. *Starting on your hands and knees, with the hands directly under the shoulders, inhale, and look up to the ceiling, lifting the chin slightly while still supporting the neck. And as you exhale, press your body back so that your tailbone is lifting behind and your chest is pressing toward your thighs.*
2. *Do your best in this position to straighten your legs by engaging your thighs fully.*
3. *Your arms should be strong and straight, with the fingers completely out-stretched, palms pressing into the floor, and the head, neck, and shoulders relaxed.*
4. *Hold this pose for 5 to 7 breaths, all the while continuing to engage the quadriceps, trying to work the heels into the floor. If at first this pose feels like too much, you can bend the knees. As you become stronger and more flexible, you will work to straighten the knees.*

INSIGHT

Push the floor away when you press up into Down Dog and spread your fingers wide apart. Bend your knees until you're comfortable in the pose, and gradually work to press your heels down to the floor. You want to keep your chest as close as possible to your thighs, and in order to achieve this position, imagine a dog as it stretches after a long nap—the stretch they do before the full-body shake. Dogs angle deeply into their hind legs as their chest moves into a deep curve hovering mere inches off the floor, a full-body stretch.

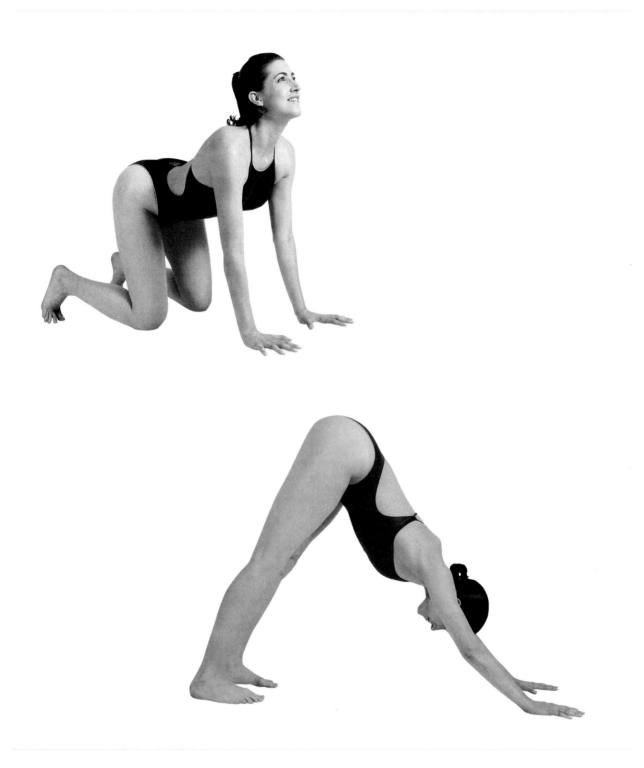

DOWN DOG NOSE TO KNEE (YOGA AND DANCE)

Strengthens all the muscles of the upper body, back, and abdominals. Increases range of motion in the hips and increases flexibility in the hamstrings, Achilles, and gastrocnemius (calf muscle).

1. *Begin on your hands and knees with the hands lined up directly under the shoulders. Inhale, and exhale to assume the Down Dog position (page 150). Arms are straight and strong and the legs are fully engaged, heels pressing into the floor.*

2. *Extend the right leg behind you, pointing the right foot about 3 inches above the floor while pressing the left heel down even farther. You should feel a stretch along the back of your left leg, starting at the Achilles and working its way all the way up to the place where the hamstring inserts into the gluteus.*

3. *Extend the right leg up even higher toward the ceiling, until you can't lift it any farther, all the while pressing the floor away with strong, straight arms.*

4. *Inhale, and as you exhale, bend the right knee, tuck the chin to the chest, and pull the navel to the spine, rounding the spine as you bring the nose to your right knee. Repeat this action 3 times: inhale as the right leg extends up to the ceiling and exhale as you tuck the chin to the chest.*

5. *After completing the last repetition with the right leg, press the right heel into the floor and repeat the exercise using the left leg. Repeat 3 times.*

INSIGHT

The trick to lifting the leg high behind you is the counterstretching and pressing you will be doing with your palms and the opposite heel on the floor. Take full advantage of the moments before you lift the leg up to enjoy the deep stretch you will feel in the back of the supporting leg. Then, after lifting the leg up behind and reaching toward the ceiling with your foot, curl the spine and tuck the pelvis under as you imagine you are a flamingo reaching its long neck down to preen the feathers on its belly.

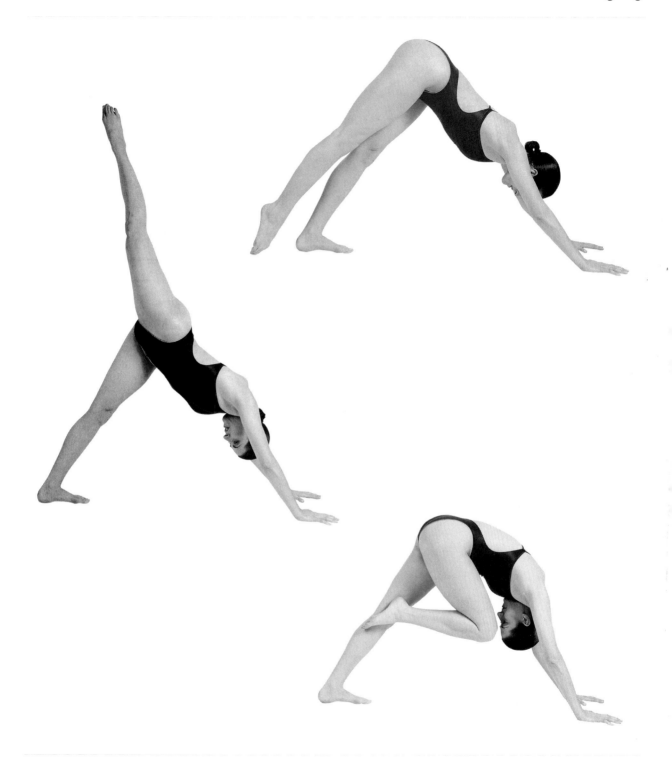

NECK PULL
(PILATES)

Strengthens the abdominals and the back. Increases flexibility in the hamstrings and lower back. A smooth, methodical exercise that asks you to move slower and slower with greater control as you do each repetition.

1. *Lie on your back in a fully extended position with the legs hip width apart, feet flexed, and arms behind the head and neck with fingers interlaced.*
2. *Inhale through the nose, and as you exhale, start to curl the upper body off the floor, bone by bone, keeping the arms behind the head and the elbows out, bringing the chin to the chest. Curl as high off the floor as possible in a* C *shape, finally bringing the forehead to the knees in a fully curved position.*
3. *Inhale as you uncurl through the spine, coming to sit up tall, with elbows open wide to the sides of the head, navel pulling to the spine. Make sure the legs are as straight as possible and the feet remain fully flexed.*
4. *As you exhale, slowly roll back down to the floor with control, one vertebra at a time.*
   Repeat 5 to 7 times.

INSIGHT

Remember to peel your body off the floor with great control. Imagine that you have your feet anchored with heavy sandbags and that your upper body leverages against this secure weight. Take advantage of the forward bending motion here and really engage the quadriceps-hamstring muscle pairing. As you roll down, engage your latissimus muscles (located slightly behind and underneath your armpits) to access greater abdominal control and move slower as you ease your body down to the starting position.

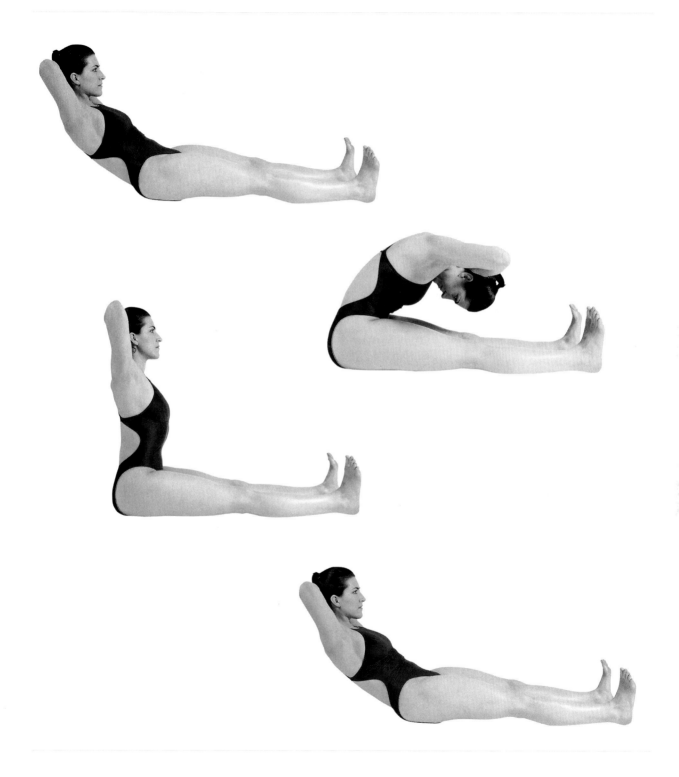

NECK PULL

ROLLOVER (PILATES)

Strengthens the abdominals, increases flexibility in the hamstrings and lower back insertions, tones the backs of the arms, and improves overall coordination while providing a deep massage for the back and internal organs.

1. *Lie flat on your back with the arms extended down by your sides, navel to spine. Bring your knees in to your chest and extend your legs straight up.*

2. *Using your powerhouse, bring your legs straight over your head so that the feet make contact with the floor behind you in a flexed position. (If you cannot touch your feet to the floor yet, take your legs only as far overhead as you are able. As you do, make sure to support the weight of your legs with your shoulders and arms.) Now open the legs to the width of your shoulders and press the heels farther back, toes curling into the floor for a stretch.*

3. *Roll down through your spine with legs still apart, one vertebra at a time, keeping the feet flexed and the thighs as close to the chest as possible. Bring your legs together in front of the body and lower them to a 45- to 65- degree angle, with feet pointed, and with control slowly take the legs back overhead to start the process again.*

4. *After repeating the sequence 5 times in this manner, reverse the movement pattern by lowering the legs down in front of you with pointed feet. Open the legs, flex the feet, and take the legs back overhead until the toes make contact with the floor.*

5. *Bring the legs together behind the head and point the feet this time as you roll the legs down past the chest back to your point of control.*
   Repeat 5 times.

INSIGHT

This is a full-body exercise that borders on being a circus trick. It is very gymnastic and requires great strength and control. Use the floor once again. It is your friend. Use it as a surface to resist and press into. You may also rely on the backs of your arms for leverage. Also very good for the kidneys and adrenal glands.

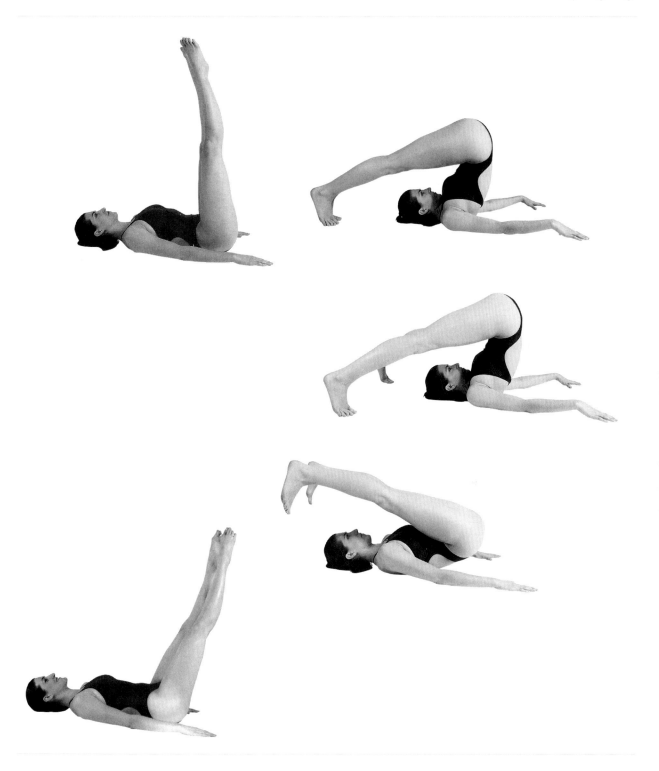

SPINE TWIST (PILATES)

Stretches the spine and the muscles of the torso, releasing tension in the shoulders and upper back. Increases range of motion in the lower back–hamstring connection. Tones the arms and conditions the abdominals and the quadriceps.

1. *Sit tall with the legs stretched straight out in front of you, heels together and feet flexed. Reach the arms behind the back, with fingers pressing against the floor so as to lift the torso higher. With the fingers pressing into the floor in this way, you will be able to establish your spine's natural curve and at the same time have leverage to lift the body higher. Roll the shoulders down and back and pull the navel to the spine. Feel the crown of the head reaching up toward the ceiling.*

2. *Extend the arms straight out in front of you. Inhale, and as you exhale, slowly reach the right hand as far behind you as you are able while continuing to lift up in the torso. You should only be twisting from your waist up. The left arm remains in front and serves as an anchor for the right side of the body, creating a feeling of opposition as you twist. Continue to exhale as your arm and waist return to the center. Make sure to empty the lungs completely on the twist.*

3. *With arms in front, inhale, and exhale as you twist again, this time reaching the left arm behind you. Remember to keep the legs straight and the feet fully flexed.*
   Do 6 sets.

INSIGHT

As you lift the navel to the spine and grow taller, engage the quadriceps so that the legs press against the floor, stretching the hamstrings. Engage your lats so that as you reach your arms in opposite directions, your shoulders will relax and you will tone your back more effectively and gain greater range of motion in the spine. Imagine that you are pressing both of your heels against the wall in front of you and that as you twist your torso, you maintain the integrity of the position. Don't shift your hips!

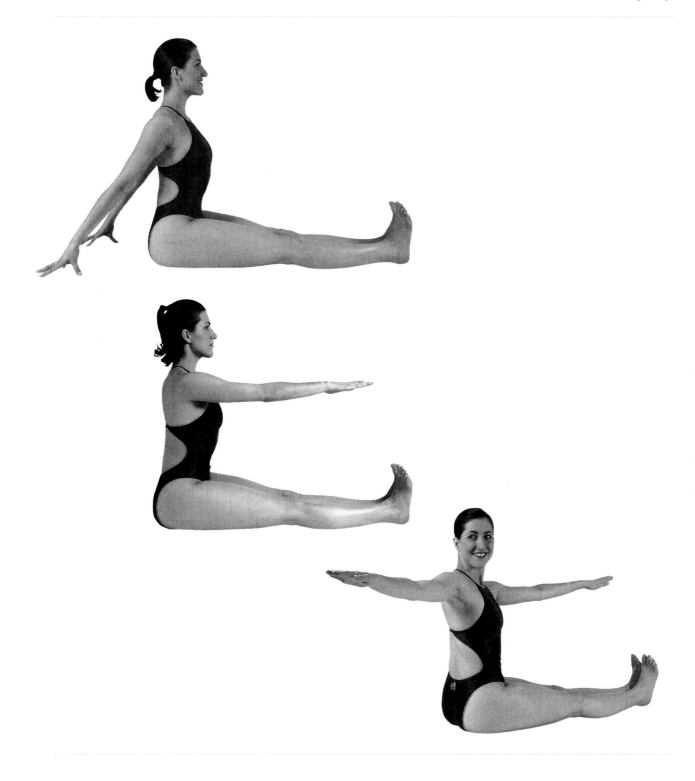

SEATED FORWARD BEND (YOGA)

This exercise is the basis for many of the seated Pilates exercises we do in this workout and will stretch and lengthen the spine and the hamstrings and promote introspection (forward bending provides the opportunity to look inward).

1. *Sitting tall with legs stretched out straight in front of you, flex the feet and make sure that the quadriceps are fully engaged. Feel the inner thighs pulling together.*
2. *Maintaining the lift in the body, reach the arms up toward the ceiling near the ears, and then start to bend the body forward, trying to maintain a straight spine.*
3. *Ultimately, with practice, you will be able to reach your toes, at which point you will bend forward as far as possible and hold the stretch for 3 full breaths. Try to be patient and know that each time you practice the exercise, you will come closer to your goal.*
4. *Repeat 2 times. The second time, intensify your lift in the first part of the exercise and then try to stretch a little farther in the forward bend.*

INSIGHT

Before you even start to fold forward, extend your torso up toward the ceiling as high as you can out of your pelvis by trying to touch the ceiling with your fingertips, and think of your fingertips as starting somewhere at your waist. Lengthen and maintain this length as you reach forward over your legs. Press the backs of your legs into the floor as you proceed, so as to stretch your hamstrings more deeply. (If you need support as you move forward into the stretch, use your hands and walk them forward alongside the body on the floor.) You may not be able to go as far forward as if you were allowing your knees to bend as they wished, but your stretch will be deeper and have longer-lasting effects.

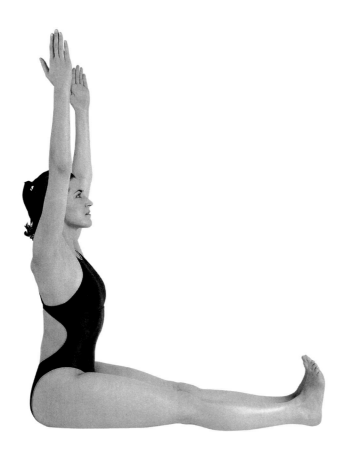

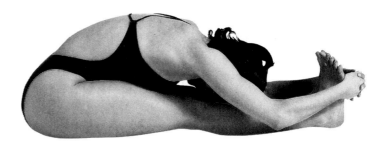

SIDE SERIES (PILATES)

One of the finest examples of the principle of opposition is the Side Series, which comprises six exercises: Pendulum, Toss-Up, Bicycle, Inner Thigh Crossover, Ronde de Jambe, and Hot Potato. It reinforces correct standing posture through core stabilization, lengthens the muscles of the legs, slims the hips, and firms the buttocks.

Some Helpful Hints for the Side Series

The body position for the Side Series remains the same throughout each exercise, with the exception of the Inner Thigh Crossover; you should assume one of the two positions shown. After executing the full series (all exercises listed) on one side, switch to the other side.

1. You can place your hand either on your mat in front of the body to brace the torso and help your control as you move through the series or on your head as you progress to the higher levels of performance.
2. Alignment for the Side Series should be as follows: elbow, shoulder, midback, and buttocks are aligned with the back edge of the mat. Legs are placed forward of the body at a slight angle (45°).
3. Make sure that the working leg is turned out, externally rotated in the hip socket.
4. Work with the principal of opposition; feel as though you are reaching your head in one direction and your legs in the other. Remember that when you establish opposition, not only do you have added stability and control, but you are creating long, lean muscles that come as a result of reaching this leg out away from the body.
5. Maintain a softly pointed foot as you work; try not to hold tension in the foot, as you want the focus of your exercises to target the upper muscles of the leg and the buttocks.

6. Always make sure that the supporting or nonworking leg is rooted to the floor and that the foot of that leg remains flexed. At first even keeping the supporting leg straight will be a challenge, but sooner than you know, you will be able to execute the series smoothly, all elements included. This is the series, perhaps more than any other, that will leave you feeling taller, longer, and leaner.

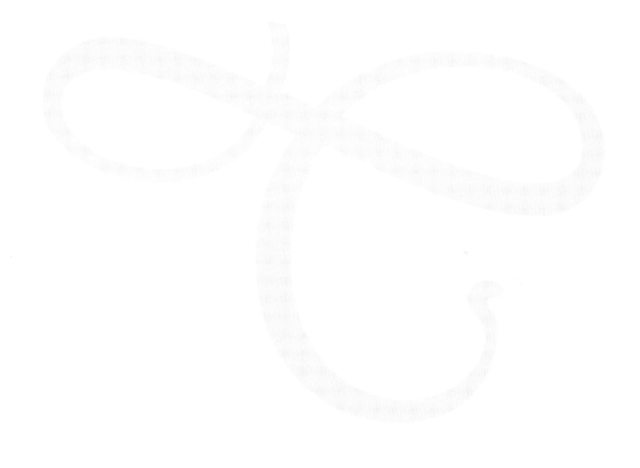

PENDULUM

1. *Lie on your right side, with the right elbow in line with the back and tail, and extend your legs at a 45-degree angle toward the front corner of your mat.*

2. *Flex both feet and raise the left leg approximately 2 inches above the right, supporting, leg. Lengthen the left foot almost as though you were going to point it; move it away from the body, assuming a soft-point position (lengthen the foot so that the toes are reaching away from the body without pointing too hard) as discussed in chapter 3, "The Nine Essential Elements."*

3. *Turn the leg out in the hip socket as though you were ultimately going to try to balance a teacup on the inside of your heel.*

4. *Make certain the navel is lifting in toward the spine, and keep the torso completely still as you proceed with the exercise.*

5. *Kick the left leg twice to the front—first a large kick, then a small kick. Swing the leg to the back with control using a similar motion: kicking it twice. Swing the leg forward again.*

6. *When kicking the leg to the front, make sure that the navel is pulling to the spine as the leg remains turned out and the torso still. When moving to the back, squeeze the buttocks for added control. (Take precautions not to let the hips rock forward or back with the leg or allow the waist to shorten; if anything, lengthen the waist and feel the lift all the way out the top of the head to reinforce the principle of opposition.)*

7. *Repeat 8 sets of the exercise, making sure to reach the leg as far away from the body as possible, always applying the principal of opposition.*

INSIGHT

In order to keep your torso still as you swing the leg front and back, imagine that you are anchored in place with two pieces of wood that are as long as your torso itself, one strapped to your front and the other to your back, which not only keep your spine and core body long and tall but also keep you still. Imagine that both pieces of wood are joined together with wide leather straps that come over your waist and are glued to you and the floor.

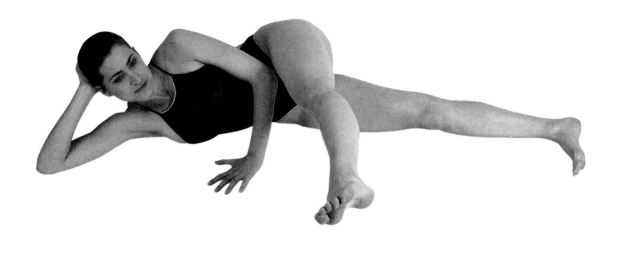

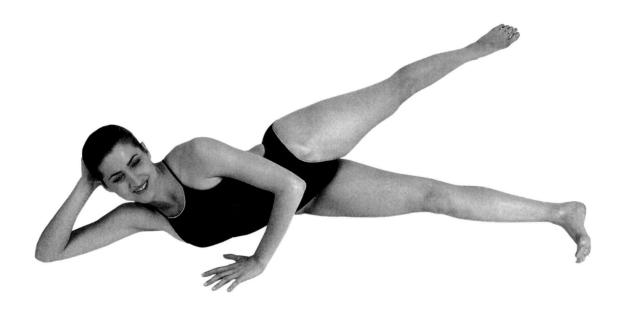

TOSS-UP

1. *Lying on your right side, go directly from the Pendulum to the Toss-Up. Point your foot and make sure the leg is rotated so the kneecap is facing up to the ceiling. Lift the left leg up as high as you can toward the ceiling. As you lower the leg, flex the foot, bringing the left heel in line with the right, supporting, heel. Remember to lengthen and strengthen at all times.*

2. *Reverse the action of the foot, flexing it on the way up and pointing it on the way down.*

   Repeat 5 times on each leg.

INSIGHT

Imagine that the ankle of your working leg is attached to a spring that is connected to the wall behind your head and as you toss your leg up to the side, the spring in the wall helps you to lift it up with the utmost control. When you bring the leg back down to line up with the supporting bottom leg, meet it with some "spring resistance" and lower it down with control. This lengthening action is really when the sculpting of the leg takes place. If you succeed in moving as though you were underwater here, you will firm the inner thigh and create real length in your quads and hamstrings.

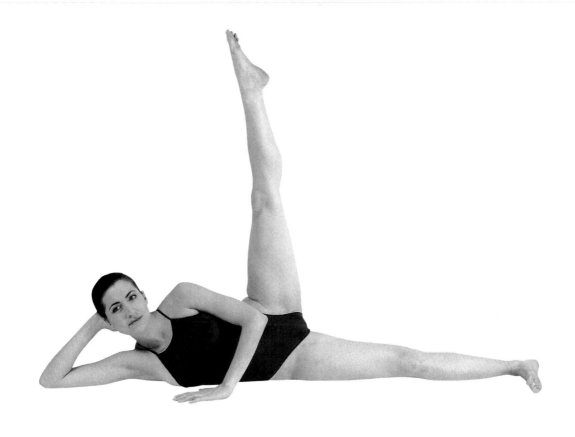

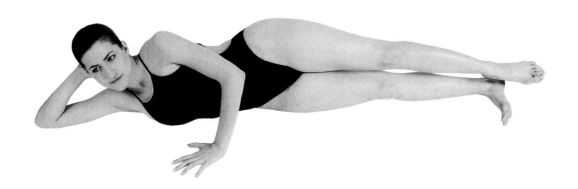

BICYCLE

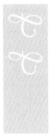

1. *Lie on your right side, with your right arm bent at the elbow, supporting your head. Lift the left leg straight out in front of the body toward your chest, using the soft point and opposition. Place your left arm in front of you, hand on the floor, for support.*

2. *Bend the left knee and bring the toe to the knee of the bottom, supporting, leg, then knee to knee, and then extend the left leg straight behind the body in an arabesque position, squeezing the gluteals and making certain that the knee is lifted completely. (As you extend the leg behind, pay careful attention to your torso, keeping the shoulders in line with one another, hips stacked, and ribs in place. It is very easy to lose control of the body here, so you must apply extra effort to your navel-to-spine connection.) Bring the leg from the arabesque position straight up to the front in a carefully controlled, flowing motion. Repeat the Bicycle 5 times.*

3. *After your fifth repetition, reverse the bicycle motion by coming back to "home," the position where the heels are stacked one on top of the other, and then take the leg back immediately again to arabesque. From this position, bend the knee and try to touch the toe to your buttocks.*

4. *Bring the knee of the working leg to line up with the knee of the supporting leg and then sweep the leg through to a full extension up toward the chest, where you first began the exercise. Repeat the reverse bicycle 5 times.*

INSIGHT

As you bring the leg to the front, try to touch it to your nose. And as you reach the leg behind, extend the leg so far out of the hip that you feel as though you could touch the corner behind you. In order to keep the leg on the same plane as it travels front and back, imagine that you are working under a large pane of glass and that you have just three inches of space above your hip, so that you don't lift the leg higher as it goes behind you, where you are not able to see it and check its position.

JENNIFER KRIES' PILATES PLUS METHOD

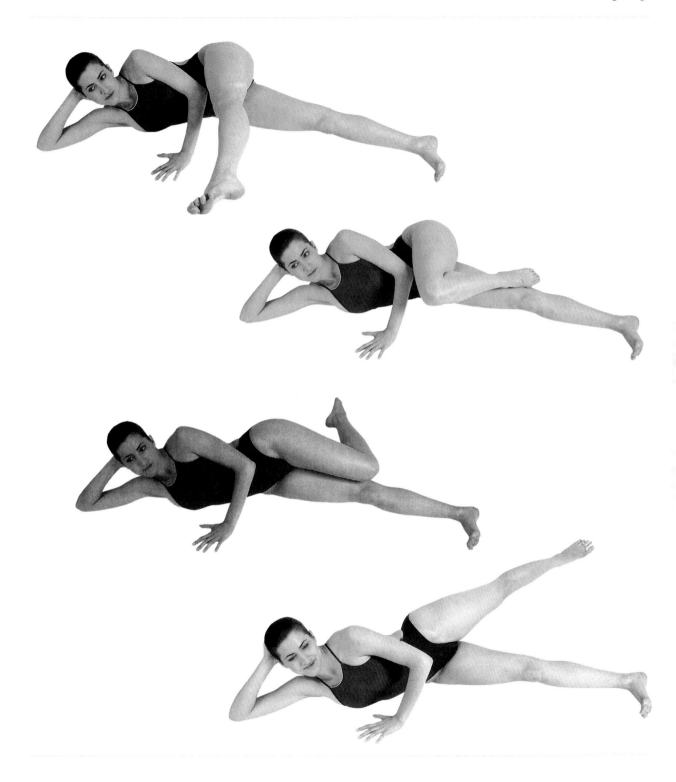

INNER THIGH CROSSOVER

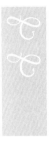

1. *Remain lying on your right side. Take hold of your left ankle and cross it over your bottom leg, placing the sole of the foot down in front of the supporting leg and torso. (If this is too awkward, you can simply place the leg on its side by allowing the knee to fall in front of the torso instead.)*

2. *With the navel to the spine, flex the bottom foot and lift the leg up as high as it will go, then lower it down with control. Don't lose the proper form in the core body; keep the hips and shoulders stacked and the neck reaching long. Repeat relatively slowly and smoothly for 10 repetitions.*

3. *After the last repetition, lift the leg one last time and circle it clockwise for 5 and then reverse the circle for 5. Finally, lift the leg as high as you can one last time and then relax it, making sure both of your heels are in alignment with each other.*

INSIGHT

Imagine that you are lifting a stack of books and balancing them on that bottom leg. Don't let the books topple from their resting spot on your leg. Remember to reach the heel as far away from the body as possible so that you lengthen the muscles of the leg as you strengthen them. Press the top, bent, leg against the thigh of the bottom, working, leg so that as you tone the bottom inner thigh, you work on increasing the range of motion in the top hip.

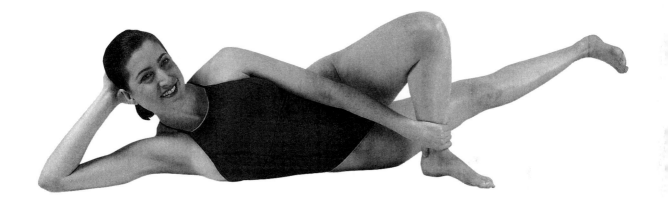

INNER THIGH CROSSOVER

RONDE DE JAMBE
(French term for the circling of the leg around the body)

1. *Lie on your right side, with your right arm bent at the elbow, supporting your head.*

2. *Take your top leg and lift it straight out in front of you toward your chest in much the same way as you did when you performed the Bicycle (page 168).*

3. *Instead of bending the leg, you will carry it straight up toward the ceiling, keeping the leg extended.*

4. *As you take the leg up toward the ceiling, have the kneecap facing up in your line of rotation—do not take the leg so high or so far to the side that you feel as though you must distort your properly placed position to achieve the side extension. Remember, height is not the issue, length is.*

5. *Bring the leg behind you and downward to the arabesque position, squeezing the gluteus for stability and allowing your hip to shift forward ever so slightly as you rotate the leg back in the hip socket. Try to reach the leg as far away from the body as possible the entire time you do this.*

6. *From the arabesque position, bring the leg back through "home," or center, and repeat the action 2 more times before you then reverse the movement sequence by starting in the arabesque position.*

7. *From the arabesque position, lifting the leg up from behind, carry the leg to the front of the body while maintaining the hips in alignment, and repeat the reverse Ronde de Jambe 2 more times.*

INSIGHT

This exercise requires real control and core strength. Pretend you have a heavy sandbag attached to the ankle of the working foot so that you maneuver the leg with grace and control through space. As you lift your leg to the front and prepare to lift it up to the side, pull the navel to the spine and adjust the hips as the leg moves from the side to arabesque behind you. You should allow your hip to shift forward ever so slightly as the leg rotates in the hip socket. In this way you will be working in harmony with your anatomical structure (in the hip and low back specifically). Use the floor for support as you sweep the leg through space in a perfect semicircle around you.

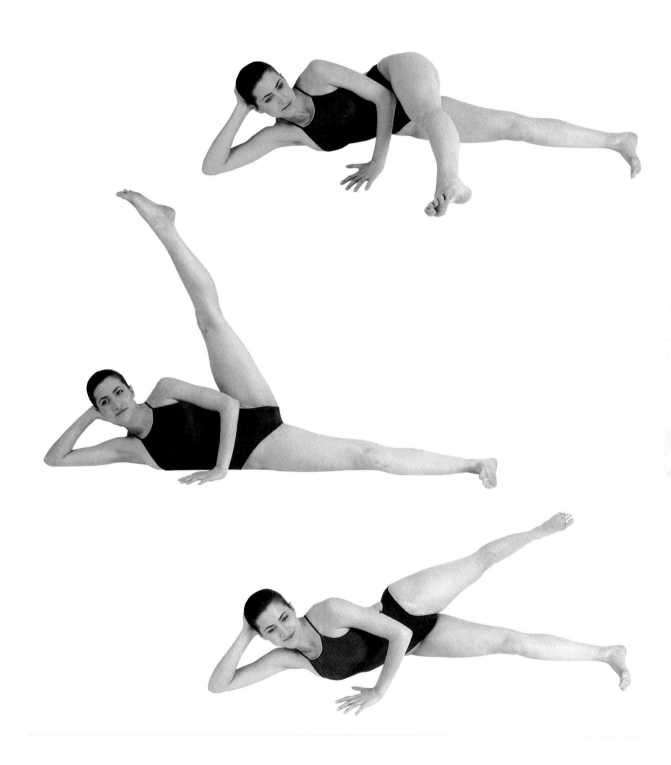

RONDE DE JAMBE

HOT POTATO

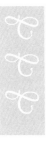

1. *Lie on your right side with your legs extended. Keeping the bottom leg still, point the foot of the top leg and lift the top leg 3 inches above the bottom one, rotated out in the hip socket. Breathe naturally and maintain the navel-to-spine connection.*

2. *Using the toes of the top leg, tap the floor lightly and quickly (with zest) 3 times with control, then lift the leg up to the ceiling as high as you can, keeping the kneecap facing up.*

3. *Sweep the leg down behind you to the arabesque position with control, and tap the foot on the floor 3 times lightly and quickly.*
   Repeat 6 times.

INSIGHT

This is a fast one! The fastest one yet, in fact. In order to stay on top of things, you must really make up your mind ahead of time that you are going to keep your core body perfectly rooted and still. As you tap the floor, know that it is the hottest surface you have ever encountered and if you linger there for more than your allotted count, you will get burned! The tempo is fast. It's front, 1, 2, 3, go! And back, 1, 2, 3, UP! The height of the leg is not important—not nearly as important as the length of the leg.

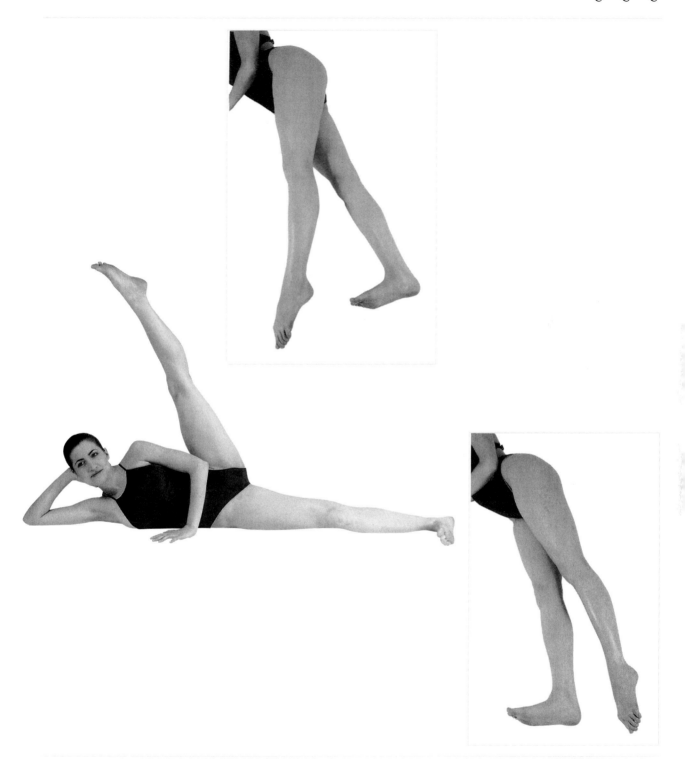

JACKKNIFE
(PILATES)

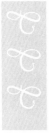

Strengthens the muscles of the back and the abdominals. Fine-tunes balance and control over the body as an integrated whole in a very advanced context.

1. *Lie on your back, legs outstretched, heels together, and feet in Pilates tripod stance (page 66). Extend your arms down by the sides of your waist, palms pressing into the floor.*
2. *Using the powerhouse, lift the legs from the floor up over the head and stretch into an angle where the legs are parallel to the floor, knees straight, toes pointing, arms continuing to press against the floor.*
3. *Reach the legs strong and straight up to the ceiling, pressing the pelvis forward from this angle, toes pointing up.*
4. *Keep the toes over your eyes as you roll down through the spine one vertebra at a time, applying the principle of opposition so as to lengthen the muscles of the legs as they extend fully down to an angle in front of the body in preparation for the next repetition.*
Repeat 5 times.

INSIGHT

The Jackknife is a glorified spinal massage and overall abdominal toner. The most important thing is to lift your legs as high as you are able to while still controlling the roll-down. Don't try to wow yourself by lifting the legs to a perfect vertical (right angle to the floor) right away, because you won't be able to roll down without lowering the legs and losing control. Choose an angle you can handle comfortably but with a degree of challenge, and then resist the roll-down by imagining that someone is pulling your feet up toward the ceiling as you roll your body, vertebra by vertebra, down into the floor.

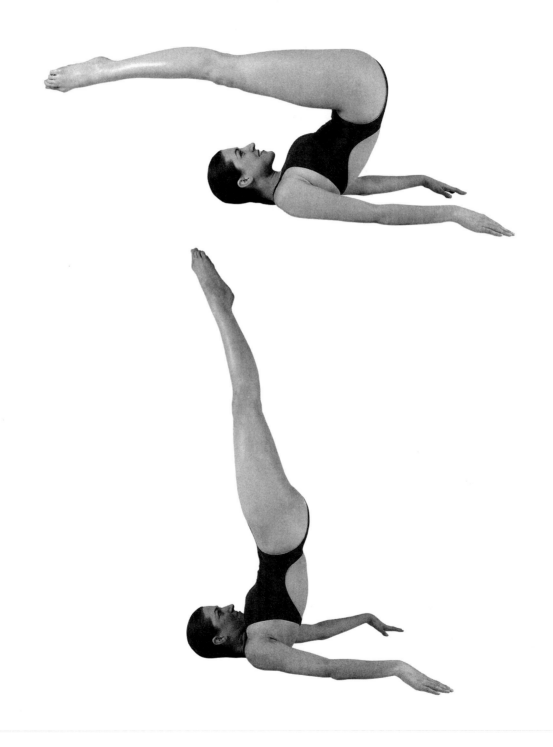

TEASER SERIES (PILATES)

The Teaser series is the benchmark of the Pilates Method. Each variation involves strengthening the abdominals against the counterweight of the extended legs. The exercises that compose the series are Single Bent-Leg Teaser, Classic Teaser, and Arms-to-Ears Teaser.

SINGLE-BENT-LEG TEASER

1. *Lie on your back, knees bent and feet firmly pressed into the floor. Lift the right leg up to match the height of the bent left knee, stretching the leg long and pointing the right foot.*
2. *Extend your arms overhead so they are stretched about 2 inches above the floor behind you.*
3. *Inhale, and as you exhale, reach your arms up to the ceiling and then toward the knees, peeling the body off the floor as high as it will go, ultimately reaching the fingers as close to the right foot as possible.*
4. *Inhale again here, at the height of the movement, and then exhale as you roll down one vertebra at a time back into the starting position.*
   Repeat 4 times using each leg.

Note: *As you become more advanced, for a greater challenge, while rolling down on your fourth repetition, bring the arms alongside the ears.*

INSIGHT

This exercise is just like the Pre-Roll-Up except that you incorporate a single raised leg. Think of pressing the foot of the supporting leg into the floor for leverage as you peel the body up off the floor and bring your fingertips toward the working foot. Imagine an electrified fence looming a foot above the floor (just under your extended leg) so that as you are working to peel the torso off the floor your working leg doesn't drop.

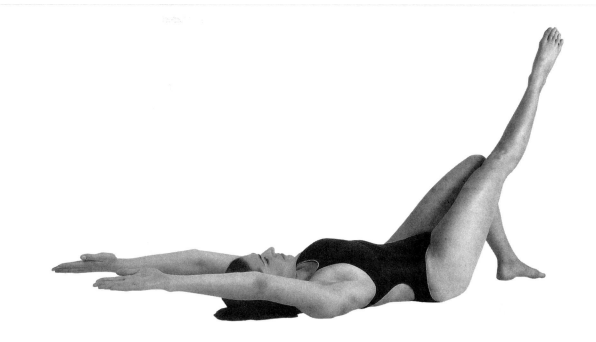

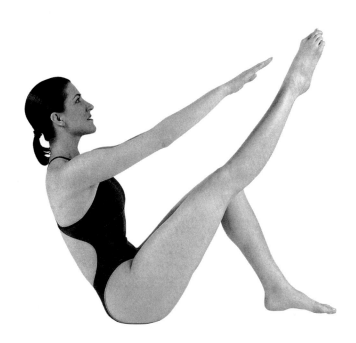

SINGLE-BENT-LEG TEASER

CLASSIC TEASER

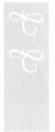

Strengthens the abdominals and the back. Firms the inner thighs and lengthens the legs. Inspires will and determination.

1. *Lie flat on your back, engage your abdominals, draw the knees to your chest, and then extend your legs straight out to your point of control (approximately a 65-degree angle).*
2. *Reach the arms overhead so that they are lifted 2 to 3 inches above the floor behind you, shoulders open and pressing against the floor.*
3. *Inhale, and as you exhale, extend fully through the legs and roll the body up off the floor with control, bringing the fingertips as close to the feet as possible without dropping the level of the legs or the lift in the spine.*
4. *Inhale once again at the height of the teaser position and exhale as you roll the body down and away from the stretched legs, vertebra by vertebra, back into the starting position.*
   Repeat 3 to 5 times.

INSIGHT

Reach your feet so far away from you once you establish your point of control that you feel as though you could actually touch the wall that lies in front of you. Apply this same effort to your fingertips, reaching them to the wall behind you; the principle of opposition will make your work much easier, creating a lightness in the legs. To ensure that your legs stay at the same level as you start to lift your upper body off the floor, put up your electrified fence and don't let the feet drop below it.

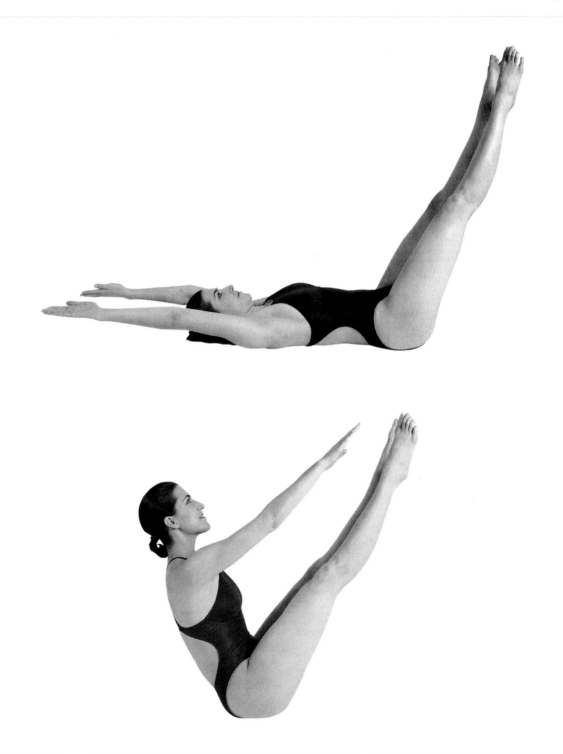

CLASSIC TEASER

ARMS-TO-EARS TEASER

Increases the challenge to the upper abdominals as the arms move to the ears, adding more weight to the upper body that the abdominals have to control.

1. *Instead of simply rolling down away from the body, lift your arms so that they come alongside the ears, and then roll down through the spine to the starting position.*
2. *You will find that bringing the arms to the ears provides you with a greater challenge, because there is then more weight that you have to contend with and control.*
   Repeat 3 to 5 times.

INSIGHT

In order to manifest the same kind of control as you did when you rolled back in the Classic Teaser, you really have to reach the legs even farther away from you (feel as if someone literally pulls your toes away from your core), providing a counterweight to your upper body, which now has more work to do with the added weight of the arms.

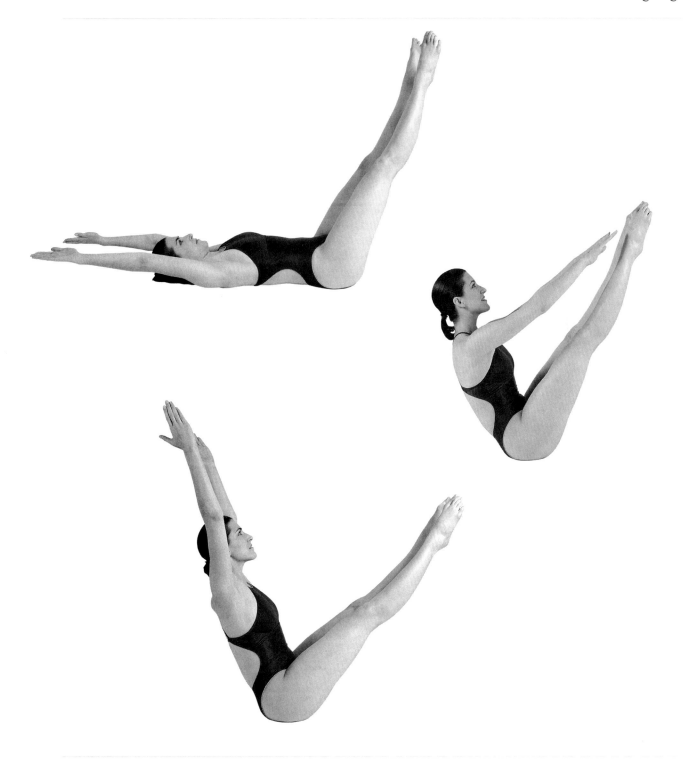

ARMS-TO-EARS TEASER

SWIMMING (PILATES)

Enhances coordination; promotes determination; tones and strengthens the muscles of the back, the hamstrings, and the buttocks. A great cross-patterning exercise (one that resembles the action of crawling, our earliest oppositional locomotive movement), an effective antidote for chronic back pain.

1. *Lie on your stomach with your arms reaching out in front of you and your legs together behind you. You should be looking straight ahead.*
2. *Reach the right arm up as high as you can off the floor in front of you and reach your left leg up behind you in the same style. Lower the right arm and left leg down to the floor with control and then lift the left arm and right leg off the floor with control. Be sure to lift your limbs as high as possible while pulling the navel to the spine and lengthening to your capacity.*
3. *Feel the opposition of the arms and the legs as you then lift all limbs off the floor; lift the head and look straight ahead as you pump the arms and the legs up and down in the air oppositionally, engaging the gluteals, the hamstrings, and the abdominals.*
4. *Continue this vigorous swimming for 20 counts, and when completed, sit back into Child's Pose (page 144) to stretch and release the lower back.*

INSIGHT

I'll run the risk of offering a rather macabre scenario here, because it makes my students laugh hard and flutter and kick really well. Imagine you are way out in the ocean, but you can still see the shore. Imagine that Jaws is after you and if you swim hard enough, lifting your legs and arms as high as you can and as quickly as you can while manifesting great control, you can escape him and make it to the shore in time.

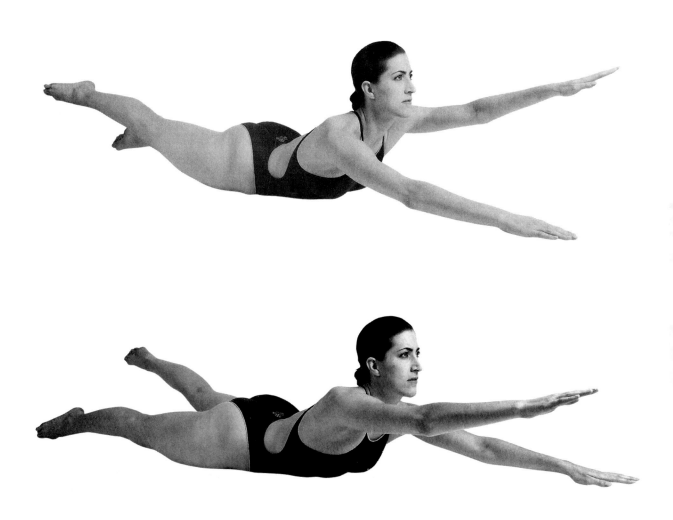

SEAL
(PILATES)

A "reward" or "dessert" exercise because it comes toward the end of the Pilates series and rewards you with a wonderful back massage. Improves coordination and balance and strengthens the abdominals as it massages the spine against the floor.

1. *Sit tall, balancing on your coccyx, with the legs open to the sides of the body in a butterfly position, knees lined up with the shoulders. Place your hands inside the legs and wrap the hands around the ankles.*
2. *Keeping the navel to the spine and the chin to the chest, clap the feet together 3 times. Using the legs as well as the abdominals, pull into the back and initiate a roll backward.*
3. *Inhale on the way back and exhale on the way up to balance. Tap the feet 3 times again as you balance on the coccyx before starting the roll back again. Repeat 5 to 7 times.*

INSIGHT

When Pilates developed this exercise, he found his inspiration at the zoo, actually observing seals as they begged for their dinner. When you clap the feet together during your balancing moments, pretend you *are* a seal balancing on its flippers and barking as you clap your entire leg and foot, one against the other.

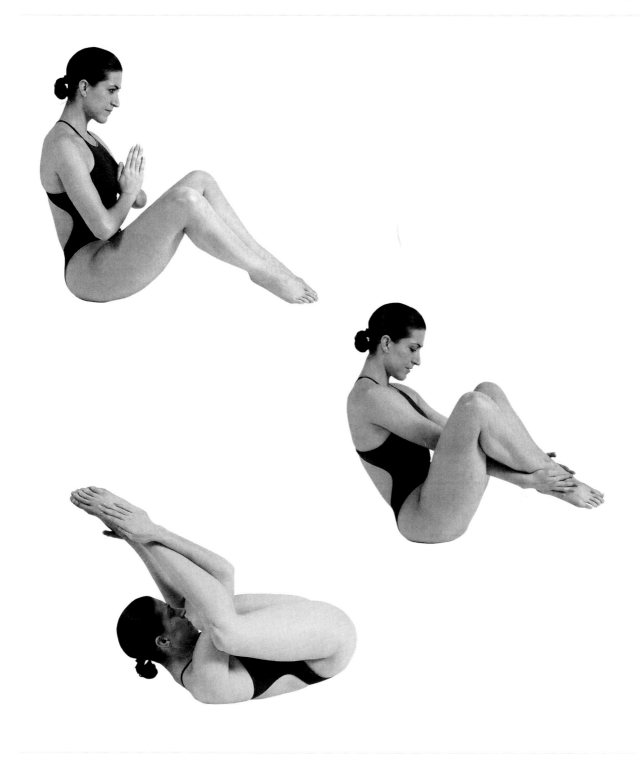

SEAL

BOOMERANG
(PILATES)

Improves overall coordination and balance. Stretches the hamstrings and strengthens the lower back and the abdominals.

One of the grandaddys of all Pilates circus-style tricks, the Boomerang is actually not as difficult as you might think. The key is to take your time and break the exercise down into its component parts when you are first learning how to do it. It combines elements from the following exercises, which you already know: Rollover, Classic Teaser, and Seated Forward Bend.

1. *Sit tall, with your legs extended in front of you, your right ankle crossed over the left. Place hands down by the sides of the hips. Inhale, and exhale as you curl the spine forward slightly, pulling your abdominals in.*

2. *Inhale as you roll the body backward, carrying the legs overhead (as in Rollover), and exhale as you continue to press the backs of the arms long against the floor. In this position, inhale and open and close the legs in a sharp and quick motion, uncrossing and then quickly recrossing, switching to the other leg on top.*

3. *Engage the inner thighs for control, finishing with the left ankle on top, and exhale as you roll up into the teaser position with the arms reaching up for the toes. Inhale as you keep the legs steady in this position, and bring the arms gracefully behind to the lower back, where you will clasp the hands together.*

(continued on page 190)

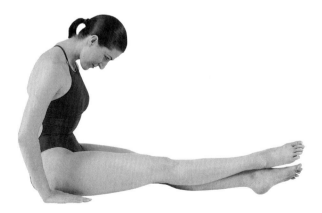

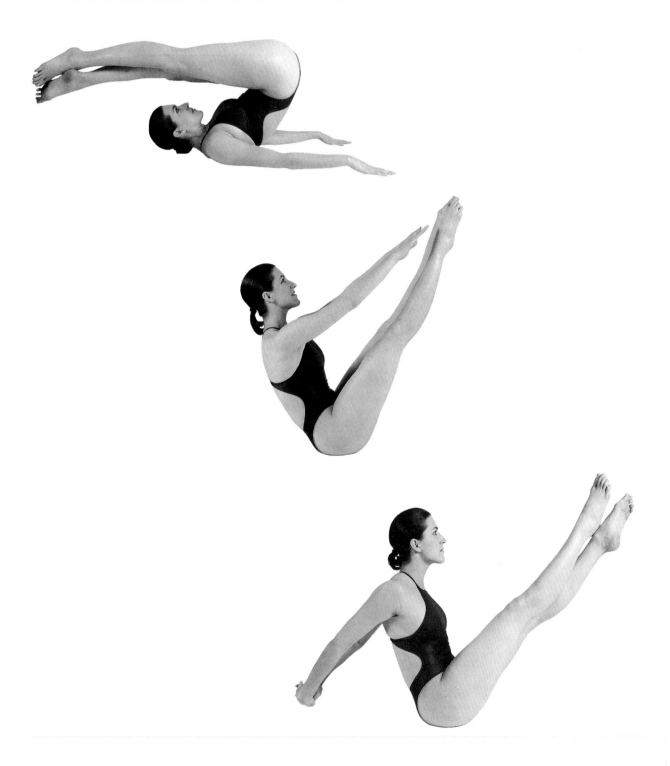

BOOMERANG

4. *Exhale as you start to lower the legs to the floor with control, shifting the pelvis forward as the arms come up behind the body. Finish with the arms up overhead, clasped behind you, with the head down as close to the thighs as possible, spine rounded forward in a C shape, with abdominals lifted.*

5. *Inhale again as you unhook the hands from their position behind the back, and exhale as you bring the arms smoothly around the sides of the body while keeping the head down toward the thighs. Finish by bringing the arms forward to the feet, where you end in a forward bend, stretching through the hamstrings.*

6. *Inhale as you roll up through the spine one vertebra at a time to your starting position.*

Repeat 4 times total.

INSIGHT

As you come up into the teaser, you can use your hands on the floor as leverage until you feel secure enough to just move seamlessly (the less you use your hands, the more you will be relying upon your core strength). As you move from the teaser to the forward bend over the legs, extend your arms as far as possible behind you in opposition away from the hips and pelvis, which you'll want to slide forward (in a sense, almost underneath you, the way you would slide a towel under a pile of clothes on a shelf). Or you can envision that someone is pulling your hips forward—the way a dance partner would pull your hips toward him or her in an embrace—as you reach your arms behind, away in opposition. If you establish an equal and opposite force, you will create the right degree of tension between the upper and lower body to move smoothly in your transition from teaser to forward bend.

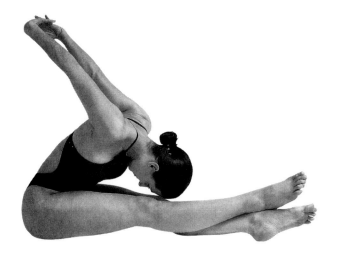

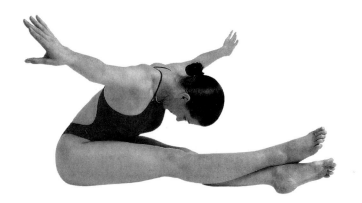

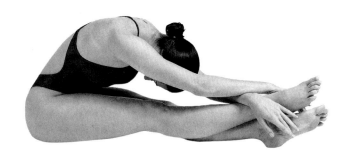

INCLINE PLANK (YOGA)

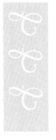

One of the most challenging upper- and lower-body strengtheners, which simultaneously opens the chest and shoulders. Improves balance and strengthens the muscles of the calves and feet. Inspires dedication and determination.

1. *Sit up tall, with the legs extended out in front of you. Inhale as you take the arms behind the body and press the hands into the floor.*
2. *Exhale and lift the center of the body up off the floor in one long plank position. Do so by squeezing the buttocks and engaging the hamstrings, lifting the hips up high (without hyperextending in the lower back) and opening the chest and shoulders to the ceiling.*
3. *Stretch the feet long against the floor, and use all the muscles of the foot to assist in supporting this lifted stance.*
4. *The first time you do this exercise, keep your eyes focused on the abdominals, and the second time, if you feel confident in the pose, you can drop your head back with control for an added challenge.*
   Do 2 times.

INSIGHT

The idea to have in mind while performing this exercise is the image of bringing your hips so high that they come to touch the ceiling. As a result, you will engage the gluteals and hamstrings and take the pressure off your arms and shoulders and center the effort in your core. Rejoice in the deep stretch you will feel, the liberating sensation of opening in your upper body, and take full advantage of the chest expansion by breathing deeply and fully, sending fresh oxygen to each and every part of your fully extended form.

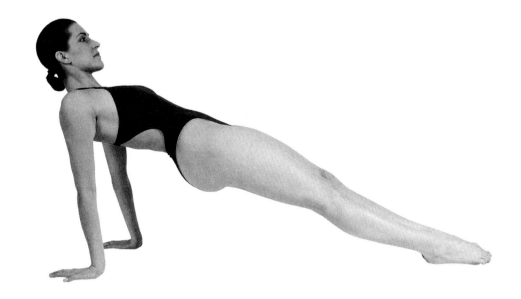

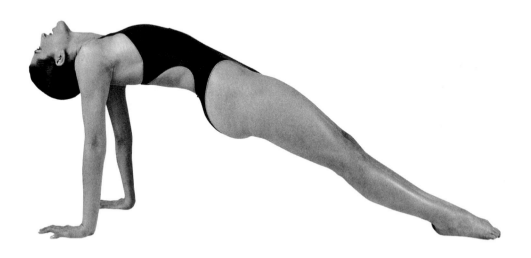

INCLINE PLANK

Strengthens the muscles of the chest, shoulders, back, and legs and stretches the hip flexors, quadriceps, and hamstrings.

1. *Stand tall with feet together in a parallel position (called Mountain Pose), and inhale as you sweep the arms up overhead, palms coming together.*

2. *Exhale and swan dive the body forward, bringing the palms to the floor on either side of the feet.*

3. *Inhale and look up, lifting the torso up slightly to a flat-back position, fingertips lengthening toward the floor.*

4. *Exhale and drop the chest back toward the knees, palms coming to the floor. Bend the knees and step the left foot back, making sure that the right knee is aligned over the foot.*

5. *Join the right foot to the left, coming into Plank Pose, where the hands are pushing the floor away, lined up directly under the shoulders, heels in line with the toes, navel to spine, buttocks tight and pelvis tucking under, creating one long line with the body.*

(continued on page 196)

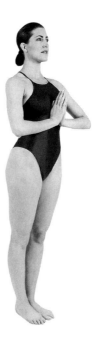
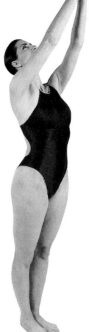

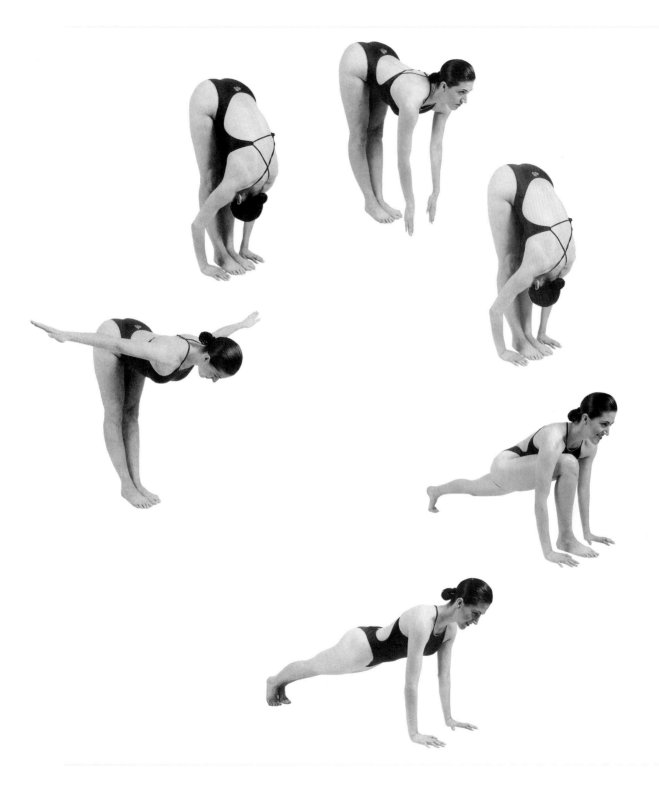

6. *Gently drop the knees to the floor, followed by the chest and chin lightly grazing the floor; the back is arched up so that the buttocks are high, and the elbows are tucked in toward the body. The arms should control the upper body as it approaches the floor.*

7. *Inhale as you pull the chest through the hands into a cobra position, chest skimming barely above the floor, lengthening the legs straight behind the body, heels together. Squeeze the buttocks tight and lift the chest, bringing the shoulder blades together, eyes straight ahead, upper back as tall as possible, with the elbows bent and tucked in to the sides of the body.*

8. *Exhale as you press your palms into the floor, extending your arms in front of you, pressing the heels into the floor behind you. Come into Down Dog, bringing your chest as close to the thighs as possible, engaging the quadriceps. Inhale and exhale here for several breaths.*

9. *Inhale as you bend the knees and step the right foot forward coming into a lunge, with hands pressed into the floor on either side of the right foot, gaze forward, left leg strong and straight behind you.*

(continued on page 198)

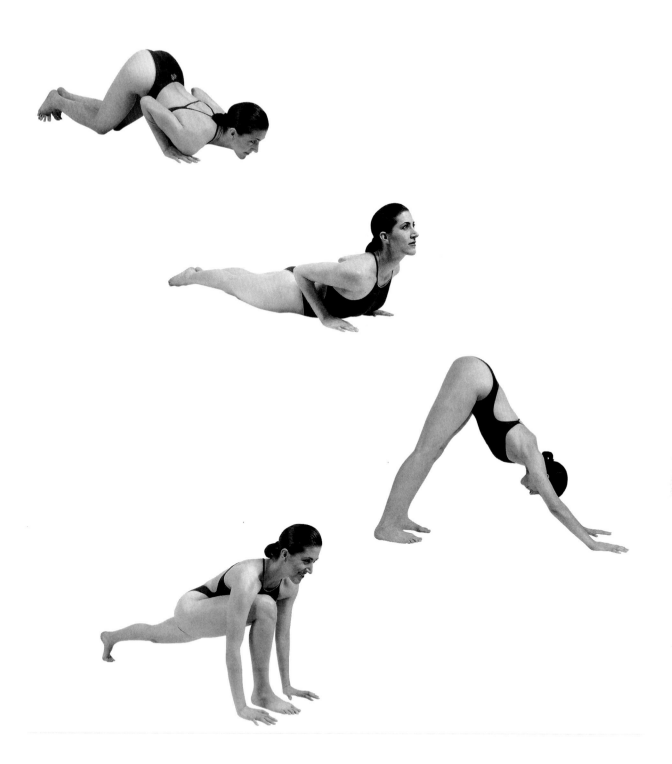

10. *Exhale and step the right foot forward to join the left, coming into forward bend with palms pressed against the floor, head down toward the knees.*

11. *Inhale and swan dive the body up, palms coming to touch overhead, then exhale and sweep the arms down to the sides of the body, coming to rest in Mountain Pose, with palms together in front of the chest.*
    Repeat the series a second time, reversing it by stepping back first with the right foot.

INSIGHT

Think of this series as a celebration. It is the first time you explore your entire body, moving from a standing posture, beginning with the sturdy Mountain Pose, to opening the arms up and around the body when you will collect the space around you (when palms come to touch overhead), to swan diving forward (deep stretch for chest, back, and legs), to a standing forward bend (a moment for introspection). When you "collect the space around you," when you go from palms together in front of the chest to arms sweeping up overhead, imagine that you are collecting snowflakes in your hands and arms as you sweep them up to meet. Really stretch your arms out far away from you.

Use the floor as a leveraging surface. Push the floor away when you go through "knees, chest, and chin folding toward the floor" into Cobra and then into Down Dog. Really spread your fingers and palms wide as you step through to lunge, and keep the images of the representative animals in your mind as you weave together the many elements you have already acquainted yourself with—the Cat-Cow, Down Dog, and Cobra. Make the animals come alive in your body; use them and their distinct movement qualities as your guide to maximize each position you move through.

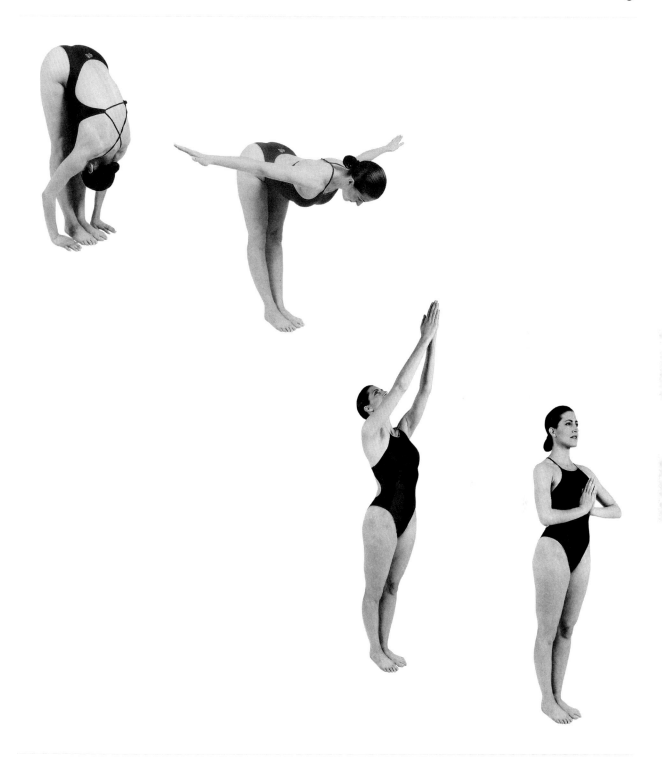

HIP FLEXOR SERIES WITH LUNGES (YOGA AND DANCE)

Stretches the hip flexors; strengthens the quadriceps, hamstrings, and gluteals. Improves coordination and balance.

Repeat steps 1 through 3 from the Sun Salutation on page 194.

1. *Exhale and drop the chest back toward the knees, palms coming to the floor. Bend the knees and step the right foot back into a lunge position, palms pressing into the floor on either side of the foot. Drop the right knee down to the floor and lift the hands onto the left knee, bringing the torso to an upright position, stretching through the right hip flexor. Breathe here for several breaths.*

2. *To intensify the stretch, bring the right arm up toward the ear and arch the upper back up toward the ceiling, allowing the weight of your torso to pull you up and back.*

3. *Curl the right toes underneath you, bring the hands to rest on top of the left knee, and straighten the right leg behind you, so as to lift the knee off the floor. Stabilize your legs and press the torso to a full upright position.*

4. *On the inhale, reach the arms up by the ears toward the ceiling. Feel the stretch in your hip flexor as you tuck the pelvis underneath you.*

5. *As you exhale, float your arms down as you bend the back knee once again to the floor. Return your hands to your left knee.*

6. *Place your palms on the floor on either side of your front foot to help you bring your back foot up to meet the front. Take a few breaths in the forward bend and then swan dive up on the inhalation to return to Mountain Pose. Repeat the entire sequence with the left leg extending behind.*

INSIGHT

Imagine you are underwater as you execute the Hip Flexor Series with Lunges. You will be able to balance more effectively and move with the control and grace that is required to execute the movements of this series. Push the floor away from you as you lift the body up from the lunge, and as you bend the knee and move down to lunge forward, feel the crown of the head spiraling up toward the ceiling so that you continue to create length in the torso as you move through the series. Think opposition!

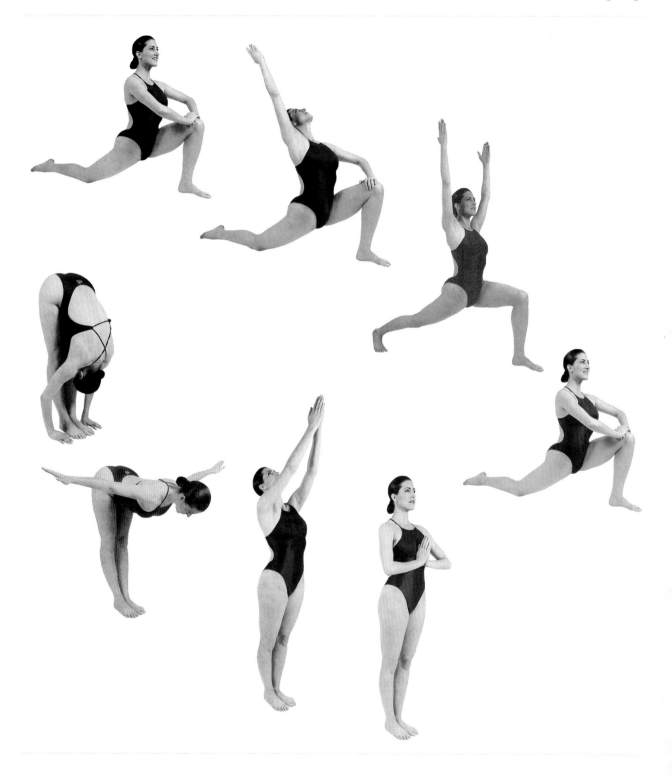

SUN SALUTATION
WARRIOR II (YOGA)

Inspires patience and mastery, creates a feeling of pride and strength for the spirit. Strengthens the legs, the upper body, and the back and creates length in the spine and in the back of the legs.

Repeat steps 1 through 3 from the Sun Salutation on page 194.

1. *Exhale and drop the chest back toward the knees, palms coming to the floor. Bend the knees and step the right foot back, making sure that the left knee is aligned over the foot.*

2. *Turn the right foot out and windmill the arms up by your sides to Warrior II. Bring the torso to an upright posture. The right arm should extend behind the body, mirroring the line of the right leg, and the gaze floats over the left arm, which is extending forward over the left bent knee. Make sure that the left heel is lined up with respect to the right foot so that it would intersect it perfectly if you were to draw a line between the feet.*

3. *Make sure that the left knee is bent as close to a right angle to the floor as possible, knee lined up directly over the foot, that the chin is lifted slightly, and that the head is held high in a proud stance, hence the name Warrior.*

4. *Hold the Warrior II position for 3 to 5 breaths and then windmill the arms down to either side of the left foot, coming into Plank Pose as in step 5 on page 194. Drop to your knees, chest and chin position coming into Cobra and then into Down Dog.*

5. *From Down Dog, step the right foot forward and reverse the Warrior II pose, bending the right knee and establishing the pose so that the left leg is extending back. Hold this pose for 3 to 5 breaths and then windmill the arms back down to the floor, where you will come into a lunge and then Plank Pose, then press down to floor and come into Cobra.*

6. *From Cobra, back to Down Dog, and then step the feet forward to come back into Mountain Pose, as follows:*

7. *Inhale and swan dive up, sweeping the arms up to palms together overhead. Exhale as you bring the arms down by the sides of the body, coming to rest finally in prayer position standing in Mountain Pose.*

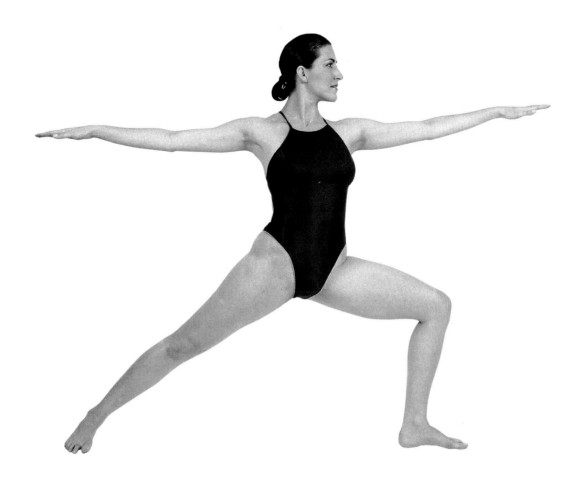

INSIGHT

Warrior II is an especially empowering pose. It is demanding and rewarding at the same time. As you go into the pose, feel as though you were growing taller in your core body (creating length in the torso through opposition again), make sure that you reach your arms in opposite directions as far as you can, and open the chest and lift your chin as you gaze with a clear, laser-beam focus over your outstretched hand in front of you, truly assuming the countenance of a proud warrior.

PLIÉ SERIES (DANCE)

And now for your crash course in ballet. The entire ballet series will shape and tone your arms, chest, shoulders, legs, hips, and buttocks. It will strengthen the muscles of the foot, ankle, and calf, as well as help with standing balance, spatial awareness, and coordination—not to mention increasing your level of integration regarding the use of your abdominal center in controlling the mechanics of your legs and arms. If you want added stability, feel free to grab on to a chair; as you gain strength and balance, you will be able to perform the series standing in the center of the room without any assistance.

First and Second Positions

First you will need to establish your turn-out line, or angle of rotation, in your hips. Stand with the feet together and parallel, shift your weight back slightly over your heels, and in one clean, controlled motion, open your toes as much as you comfortably can, making sure your knees are in line with your toes. Don't readjust this "natural" position your body has just found for your feet. You want a manageable line of rotation so you can work safely and effectively and at the same time maintain the integrity of your turn-out (knees over toes and knees in line with the hips).

FIRST POSITION

1. *Push the floor with your feet and reach the crown of your head up toward the ceiling, lengthening behind the neck and through the length of your spinal column. At the same time, squeeze your buttocks and pull the abdominals in for added control.*
2. *Lift your arms out from the sides of the body. Lift up the elbows, imagining you are hugging a big beach ball. Gently shape the hands as though you were gracefully holding a teacup in each one.*
3. *Bring the arms together in front of the body to form a complete circle in front of the chest; take a deep breath in, and exhale as you bend the knees over the toes while keeping the heels rooted to the floor. Sweep the arms*

down toward the hips and open up and out to the sides where they began. This action is called plié with port de bras (arms).

4. *From the bent-knee position, inhale to come back up to the starting position, where the legs are fully engaged, kneecaps lifted, buttocks squeezed tight, and the arms are forming that circle in front of the chest, where you will begin the process again and repeat 4 times total.*

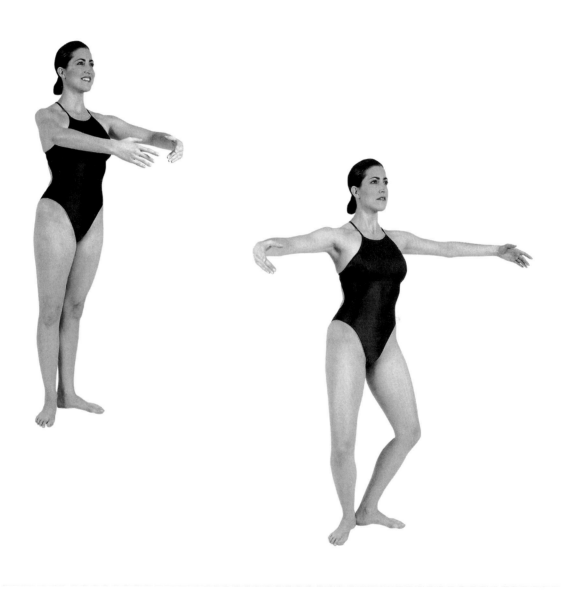

SECOND POSITION

1. *For second-position pliés, you will repeat the same steps as in first position, but before you begin, shift the weight slightly over the left foot, with arms out to the sides for balance. "Tendu," or fully stretch the right foot, opening it to the side of the body, where it will come to rest. The right foot should lie flat and in line with the left foot. Now you are ready for second-position pliés.*

2. *Make sure that the knees are in line with the feet as you bend them, as far as your Achilles tendons will stretch. Keep the heels rooted to the floor. The arms will sweep through the exact same positions as in first-position pliés.*

INSIGHT

For the upcoming ballet exercises, the arms will remain either up in front of the body or to the sides throughout, the buttocks should be fully engaged at all times, chest lifted, eyes high, spine tall. During the series, think of pushing the floor and the ceiling away with your feet and head as you straighten the legs between knee bends. As you lengthen into a tall, straight standing position, and as you descend into a plié, continue to reach up out of the crown of your head, again envisioning the barber shop pole spiraling upward. See the roots of the tree anchoring into the earth below.

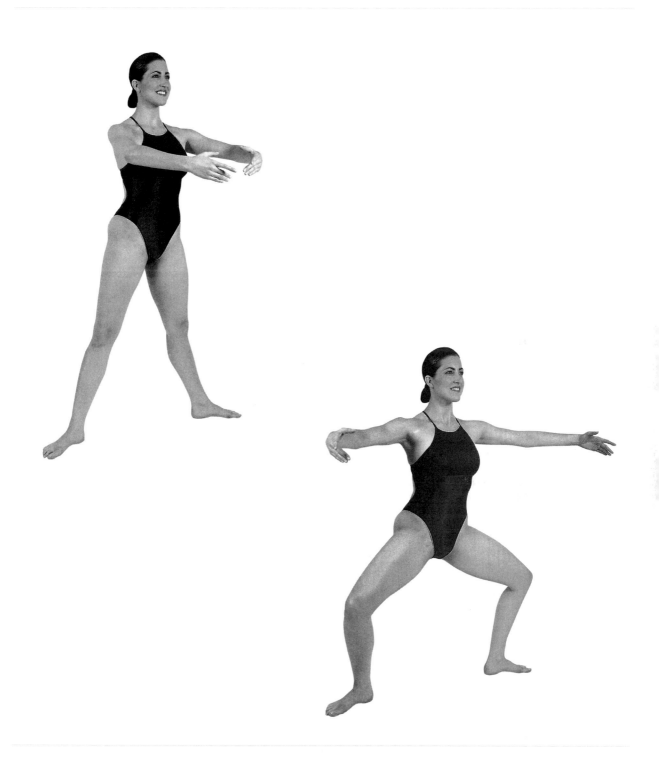

SECOND POSITION

207

TENDU EN CROIX

1. *Stand in first position. Shift your weight slightly over the left foot and lift your arms up and out to the sides. The arms will remain out to the sides throughout the exercise.*

2. *Starting on the right, brush the foot against the floor and point it fully so that all the muscles of the foot are directed to a place on the floor in front of the body that lies directly in your line of rotation down the midline of the body (in line with your nose or belly button).*

3. *While the foot is pointing in tendu, all the muscles of both the working leg (in this case your right) and the supporting leg are engaged. All the muscles are stretching, with the energy directed through the toes to the floor.*

4. *Bring the foot back toward the left heel to return it to its starting position by initiating with the baby-toe side of the foot first to maintain your turnout. Press the ball of the foot, then the arch, and then the heel against the floor as you sweep it back in an arclike motion to meet the left heel. Repeat the tendu 3 more times to the front before moving on to the side and the back.*

5. *To tendu to the side, start from first position and point the foot to the side in your line of rotation, applying the same mechanics as you did to the front. Make sure that when you bring the foot back to first position, you engage the inner thigh to initiate the action.*

6. *When you go to tendu to the back, or arabesque, the most challenging of all the positions so far, allow your body weight to shift even more to the left foot and toward the front, so that as you move the foot back, you gently arch your back and accommodate the transfer of weight by shifting forward slightly in your pelvis, pressing the hips forward.*

7. *When you point the foot to the back, make sure it goes directly behind you, toward the middle of the back. Stretch all the way through the right big toe, taking care not to press any weight against the floor. Engage the abdominals, expand the chest, and lift your gaze up slightly so that you employ the principle of opposition to lift away from the point of focus, which, in this case, is the right big toe. Extend your opposite arm up into an arabesque position in front of you as you tendu to the back.*

8. *To return to the starting position, initiate with the right heel, dragging the right ball of the foot and toes in to first position last in order to maximize the movement and use of your muscles. Repeat the tendu 3 more times to the back, and do 4 additional tendus to the side before switching to tendus on the left.*

INSIGHT

To do an effective tendu, really brush the foot against the floor with considerable resistance. Imagine that you are moving against water with your foot, brushing the foot against the bottom of a pool to move it forward or to the side or backward to a point. Then use resistance again to bring the foot back into first position. This exercise will tone the inner thigh and strengthen all the intricate muscles of the foot.

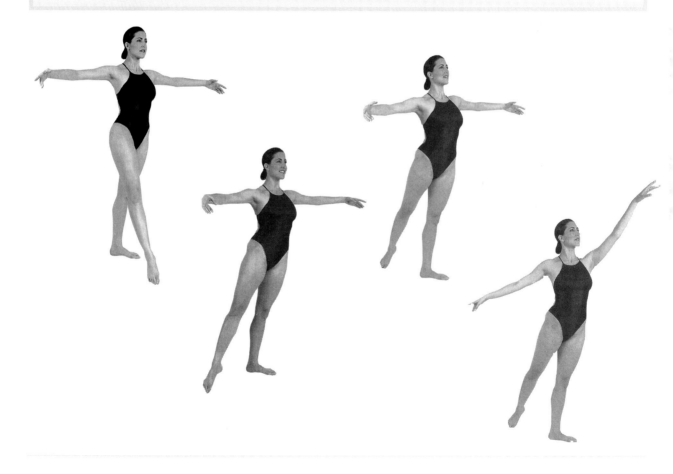

DÉGAGÉ

The nice thing about dégagés is that they are exactly like tendus, but instead of keeping the toes connected to the floor the entire time, you brush the toes slightly off the floor at the end of your extension.

1. *Start standing in first position as you did with the tendus (in your natural line of rotation), and point the right foot to the front, brushing it slightly off the floor at the end of the movement.*

2. *To bring the foot back to starting, lead with the baby-toe side of the foot and brush the foot back to first, engaging your inner thighs to initiate the return. Perform the dégagé 4 times each to the front, to the side, and to the back, applying the same principles as in the tendu series to the front, side, and back, and of course, always repeat the side again before switching to the other leg.*

INSIGHT

Try to feel as if you were pushing your foot through the sand on the beach, moving with great resistance. When you start to bring the foot back to first position (as in a tendu), lift the toes, the arch, and then the heel of the foot in one swift motion and then fully extend the foot by reaching all the way through the leg. Focus all of your body's effort on that one small point, reaching through the big toe.

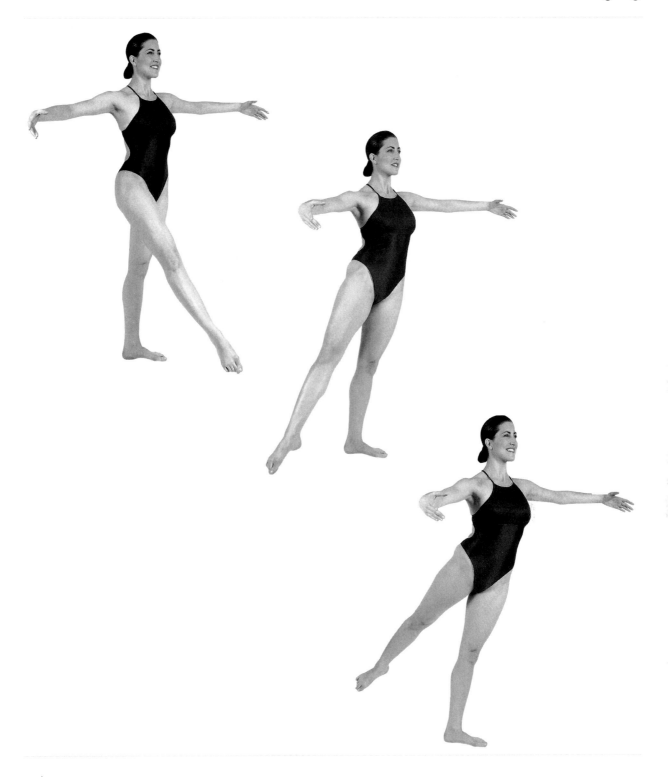

DÉGAGÉ

FONDU

1. *Start in first position and bend the knees, shifting your weight slightly to the left foot, arms sweeping down in front of the hips to come together in a closed circle, with the fingertips barely touching.*

2. *Peel your right foot up off the floor, pointing it as it comes in toward the spot just 2 inches above the left ankle, and glue it to that spot above the ankle temporarily in a fully pointed position with the right knee turned out to the side. The arms come up to form a circle in front of the chest.*

3. *From this place where both the right and left knees are bent and the right foot is pointed and glued above the ankle, performing both actions simultaneously, start to straighten the supporting leg as you extend and straighten the right leg out in front of the body in a turned-out position, imagining that you could balance a teacup on your heel.*

4. *You will come to achieve a position that looks exactly like dégagé to the front, where both legs are straight and the arms have gone from their position down in front of the hips up through their place in front of the chest, finishing out to the sides where they began.*

5. *From the extended position to the front, bring the right leg into the plié position (legs turned out in their natural line of rotation) again, pointing the right foot all the while, as you bend the left supporting leg simultaneously and bring the right toes back to that spot just 2 inches above the ankle.*

6. *From here you will extend both legs simultaneously again, repeating the sweeping pattern with the arms, this time taking the foot out to the side, pointing it completely and fully extending through both the supporting and working legs.*

7. *Keeping in mind the principles that you applied to dégagé to the back, bend the knees again, and this time bring the toes behind the supporting ankle and extend the leg to the back in arabesque. Make sure that you direct the leg to go exactly behind the body, aiming for the opposite shoulder.*

You will simply perform 1 fondu in each direction, unlike tendu and dégagé.

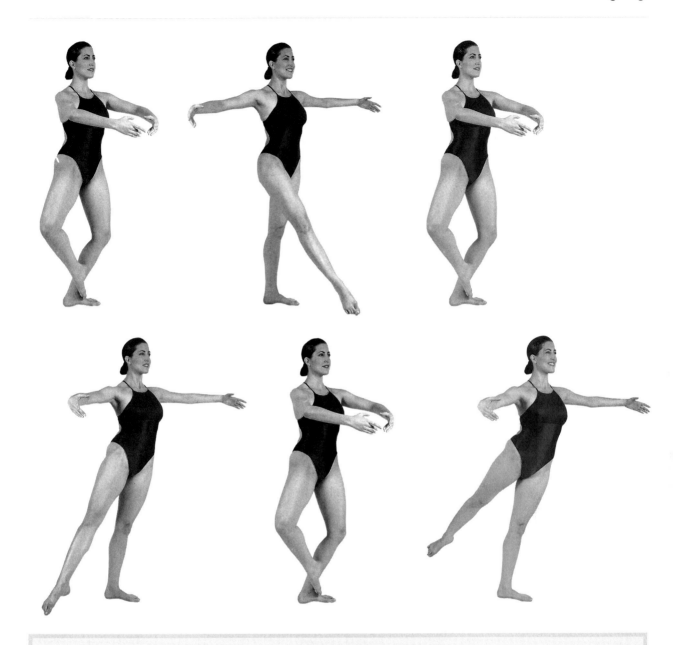

INSIGHT

As you bend both knees in the fondu, feel as if you are melting (hence the name), even though you continue to reach through the crown of the head toward the ceiling in opposition, all the while applying the utmost control and grace to your movements.

90-DEGREE FRONT PRESS FORWARD

The Standing Sculpting Series—90-Degree Front Press Forward, Strongman, Side Bend, Chest Expansion, Boxing, Shaving the Head, Hug, and Arm Circles—strengthens and sculpts the muscles of the arms, back, chest, and shoulders, as well as the lower body, including the legs, hips, and buttocks. It improves balance and coordination and spatial awareness. All the exercises reinforce good posture and correct alignment.

Using handheld 3- to 5-pound weights (optional), hold the body in a fully upright, engaged tripod stance that helps establish correct posture and tone the entire body. The legs, abductors, and buttocks are used as a central support for the upper body. This series of highly effective sculpting exercises improves upper-body strength and definition. When you perform the exercises, apply self-imposed isometric resistance with your every movement. You may want to position yourself in front of a mirror so that you can check your alignment and observe the almost immediate change that will take place in your arms as you sculpt them.

1. *Stand tall with heels together and toes apart (tripod position). Lift the arms, with weights in hand, in front of the body so that the elbows are bent and form a right angle, palms and weights directly in front of the face. Pitch your body weight forward slightly over the toes and don't give in to the tendency to sink into your lower back. (You may want to over-compensate a little when you begin by leaning the body forward farther than you think you should.)*

2. *Squeeze the buttocks and engage the front of the thighs. Inhale as you extend the forearms, just to the place before your elbows lock. As you exhale, pull the forearms back toward the body with self-imposed resistance to the original starting position.*
   Repeat 7 to 10 times.

As you are lowering and raising your forearms, imagine you are pushing and pulling two hundred pounds. This will create the self-imposed isometric resistance you require to make your movements more effective. Additionally, don't lose sight of the fact that as you sculpt your upper body, you are also toning your lower body by continuing to squeeze your buttocks and inner thighs throughout the exercise.

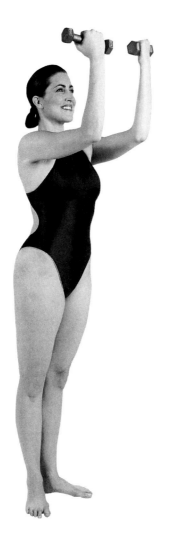
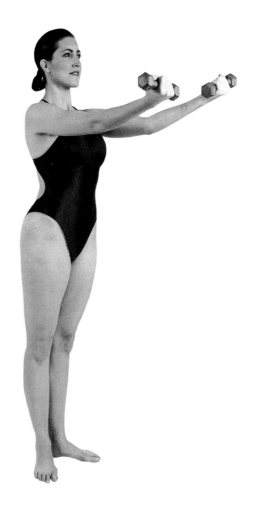

STRONGMAN

1. *Stand tall, with heels together and toes apart. With weights in hand, lift the arms up and out from the shoulders to the sides of the body, with the elbows bent again at a right angle. (Make sure they are positioned slightly in front of the body so they can be easily viewed with your peripheral vision.)*

2. *Inhale and extend the forearms away from the body just to that place before the arms lock. Feel as though you are pushing a heavy weight. As you exhale, bring the forearms back toward the body curling the hands in toward the ears with resistance.*

   Repeat this 7 to 10 times.

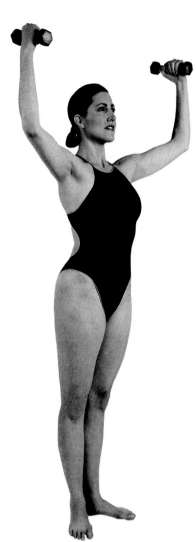

Again, use the image of pushing and pulling two hundred pounds to create the proper degree of resistance in your movements. The Strongman is a fun opportunity to play with the notion of "bodybuilder."

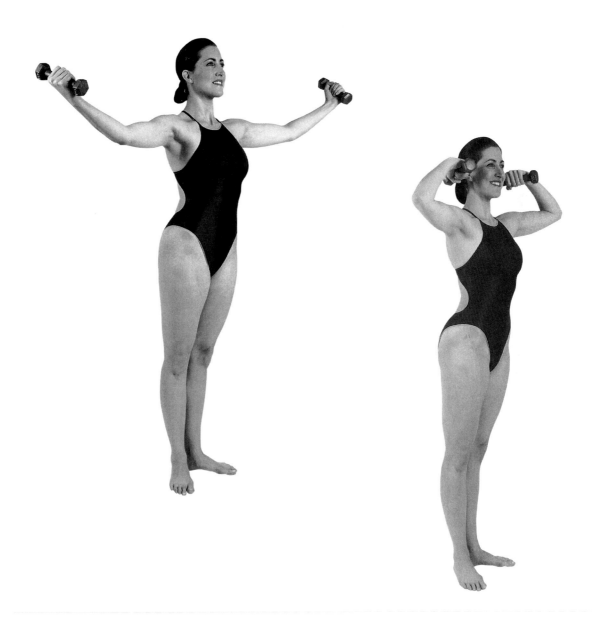

SIDE BEND

1. *Take a moment to "shake the legs out" before you do this exercise, then grab your weights (optional) and assume the heels-together, toes-apart position and lift the left arm straight up—the hand is reaching as high up to the ceiling as possible. Glue the arm to your left ear and make sure that it stays there as you continue through the exercise.*

2. *Inhale, and as you exhale, pull the navel to the spine, squeeze the gluteals, and extend the hand even higher to the ceiling as you reach the torso over to the right in a tall side bend. Allow the right hand to lengthen down to the floor as much as possible, intensifying the stretch in the side.*

3. *Inhale from the side-bend position to come back up and immediately lower the left hand with control and repeat the action, this time raising the right arm, bending to the left side. Make sure that you are not hyper-extending the ribs (allowing the ribs to stick out) and that you apply added effort to engaging your abdominals and buttocks in order to support the side bend and protect the back. Do 3 sets for a total of 6 side bends.*

INSIGHT

Apply the principle of opposition! When you lift the arm up before you do your actual side bend, try to touch the ceiling and root your lower body into the floor. Press that right foot firmly into the floor and you'll feel the stretch radiate all the way through the leg and your upper body. As you bend to the side, make sure that your chest is slightly in front of the hips so that you protect your lower back as you side bend. Squeeze your inner thighs and buttocks to stabilize your lower body.

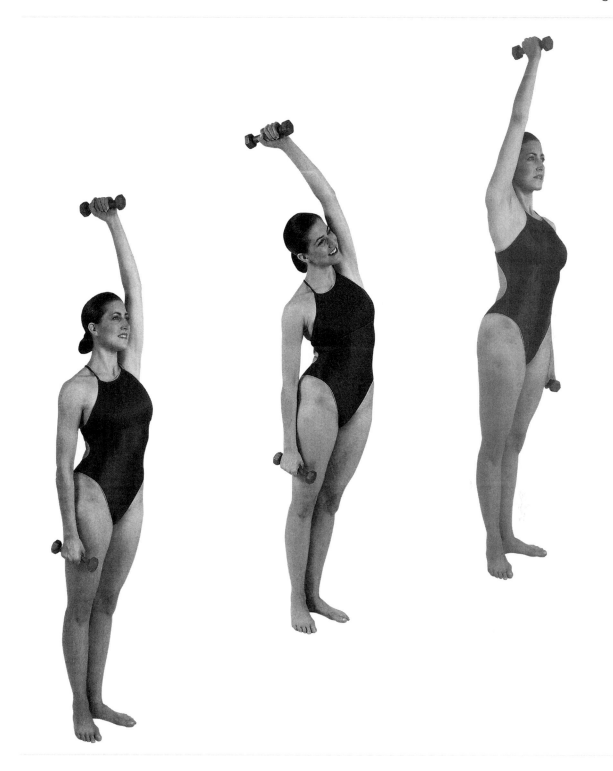

SIDE BEND

CHEST EXPANSION

1. *Stand with heels together and toes apart, buttocks engaged, navel pulled toward the spine. With weights in hand, extend the arms up in front of the chest directly out from the shoulders.*

2. *Inhale and hold the breath as you extend the arms behind the back, lifting them as high as possible, expanding the chest, squeezing the shoulder blades together, shoulders down.*

3. *Look to the right, center, and then left, maintaining the arms high behind the back, wrists as close together as possible, and then exhale as you bring the arms back up to the starting position, high in front of the chest, in line with the shoulders.*

4. *Repeat the action, turning the head first to look left, then center, and then right. Do 4 sets.*

INSIGHT

When you inhale and reach your arms behind you, fully expand the chest and lift your chin proudly—you'll feel your lungs thanking you for the opportunity to take in more air, to grow larger and fuller than usual.

Imagine you are lifting your arms underwater and envision a large sea sponge between your arms that you need to squeeze gently each time you reach your arms up behind you, providing the resistance between the arms that will engage the head of the triceps, toning the backs of the arms.

A great breathing exercise, Chest Expansion is truly an expansion, not just for the chest and shoulders, but for the lungs and heart—and for the spirit!

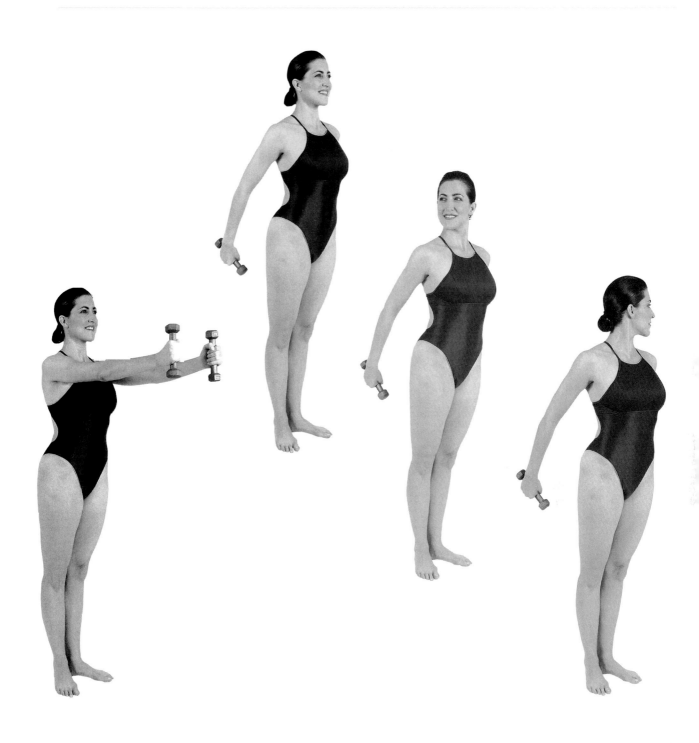

BOXING

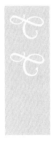

1. *Stand tall in parallel position with feet hip width apart; bend the knees over the toes and bend forward so that the torso assumes a flat-back position, with the crown of the head lengthening away from the tailbone.*

2. *Bring the hands in front of the shoulders, elbows bent, and pull the navel to the spine.*

3. *Inhale, and as you exhale, extend the right arm straight ahead, out from the shoulder, and the left arm behind the body. Continue in exactly this way, switching the arms so that the left arm reaches frontward and the right arm lengthens to the back, working the triceps and the deltoids and muscles of the back.*

4. *Inhale and exhale as you switch the arms, and make sure that the knees are sufficiently bent and lined up over the toes. Repeat 8 to 10 times. After completing boxing, round the chest forward over the thighs to release the spine, and roll up one vertebra at a time, allowing the arms to hang heavily as you roll up, making sure that the head is the last thing to arrive.*

INSIGHT

In order to create the resistance the exercise requires, imagine that you are moving the weights front and back underwater. This, by the way, is a great exercise for skiiers, as it conditions and strengthens the body in a simulated skiing posture.

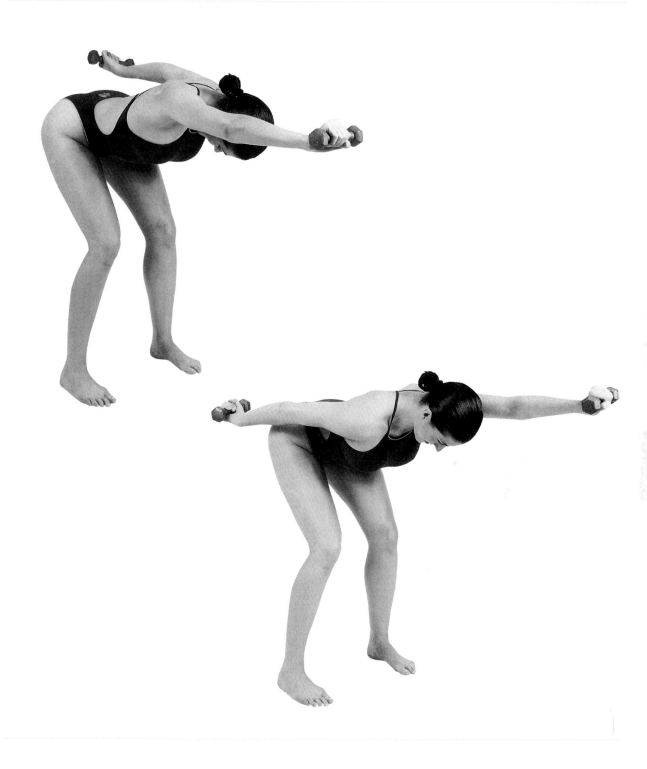

BOXING

SHAVING THE HEAD

1. *Stand with heels together and toes apart (the Pilates stance, or tripod). Raise the arms behind the head, with the elbows wide to the side, and extend the fingertips that aren't encompassing the weights so that they are just touching, or simply form a triangle if you choose not to use the weights.*

2. *The upper body is pitched slightly forward, and as you inhale, pull the navel to the spine.*

3. *On the exhalation, extend the arms straight above the head, weights still touching. Bend the arms and return to the starting position, closely grazing, or "shaving," the back of the head.*

   Repeat 7 to 10 times.

INSIGHT

Feel as if you were forming an umbrella with your hands as you reach the arms up at the angle overhead. When you bring the arms back behind the head, make sure to go through the motion of literally "shaving" the back of the head by brushing the back of your head with your hands.

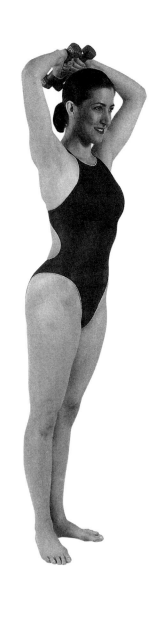

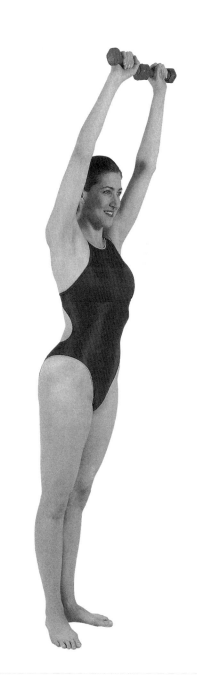

SHAVING THE HEAD

HUG

This exercise targets the deltoids and reinforces the latissimus/trapezius connection.

1. *Standing tall in tripod stance; with weights in hand, hold the arms out to the sides of the body, with the elbows lifted. Imagine you are hugging a very large beach ball.*
2. *Inhale and squeeze the arms together with resistance, feeling as though you were pulling springs toward the body, bringing the hands to nearly touch.*
3. *As you exhale, open the arms with resistance as though you were pushing very heavy weights away from the body. Perform the Hug 3 times, inhaling as the arms come together, and then repeat the Hug, reversing the breath by exhaling as the arms come together.*
Perform the Hug a total of 6 times.

INSIGHT

The latissimus-trapezius muscle pairing is really important here. Your shoulders should be relaxed as you concentrate on sculpting your upper body. Feel as though you are squeezing a huge rubber beach ball between your arms as they come together so that you work with a considerable degree of resistance. As you open your arms, create the same resistance, imagining that you are pushing two hundred pounds away. Pull the navel to the spine, squeeze the gluteals, and grow taller as you "hug" the beach ball.

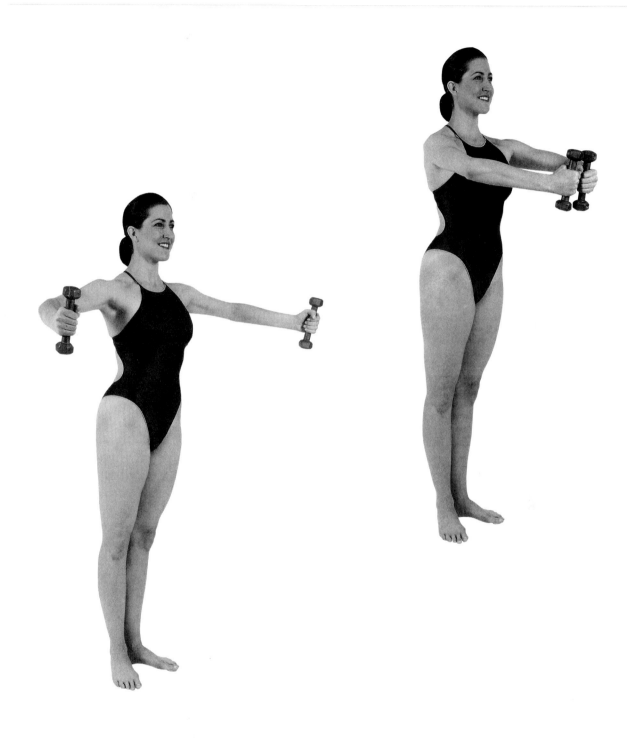

HUG

ARM CIRCLES

Strengthens the core and muscles of the back and upper body.

1. *Stand tall in tripod stance, with weights in hand, arms down by the sides. Holding the torso strong, circle the hands away from the body in small movements, working your way up to a V position above the chest.*
2. *The circles are small, concise, and strong and require that the body be held perfectly still. Circle 5 times to the up position and then 5 down. Inhale in a smooth, continuous fashion as the arms circle up and exhale as the hands circle down.*
Do 3 sets.

To make Chest Expansion, Shaving the Head, and Arm Circles more advanced, come up to a relevé (standing on the balls and toes of the feet, lifting the heels) position each time you exhale and lift the arms into position (that is, in Shaving, come to relevé when you extend the arms into their overhead position; in Chest Expansion, when the arms extend behind; and in Arm Circles, when the arms reach their highest position). Bring the heels tightly together, squeeze the buttocks and engage the inner thighs, lifting up so that all ten toes form a platform.

INSIGHT

Concentrating on keeping your core strong is the most important aspect of this exercise. Try not to move your body at all as you circle the arms upward or as you bring them back down. This exercise also moves at a slightly faster tempo than the other exercises in the Standing Sculpting Series, so you have yet another challenging component to contend with. A faster tempo involving a wider range of motion means that you have to apply extra effort and focus to your core—using the principle of opposition.

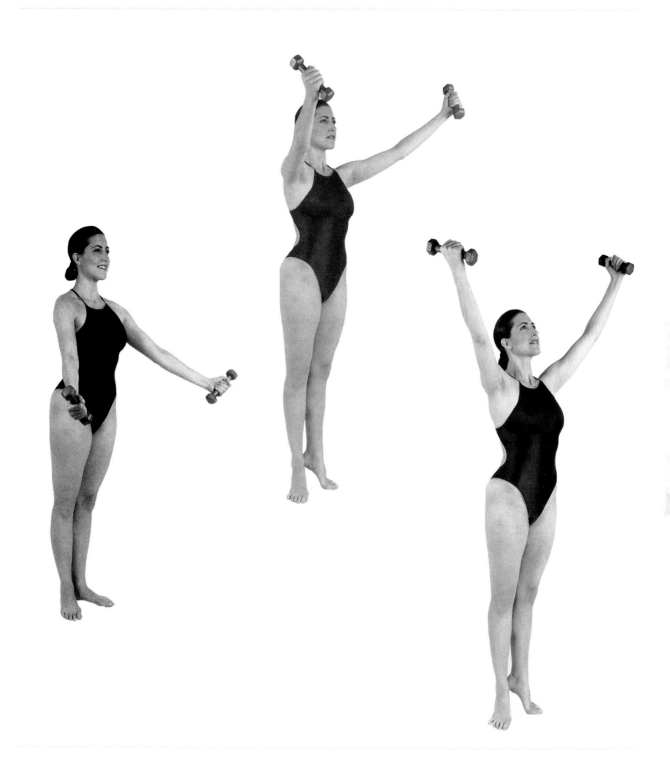

Post-Sculpting Relaxation

After completing the entire Standing Sculpting Series, you may lean your back against a wall, standing with your heels together and toes apart about 3 to 4 inches away from the wall in tripod position, and roll forward halfway so that your hands fall in line with your knees. Allow the weights to pull your hands down and relax your arms in their shoulder sockets. Let gravity help you as you make tiny circles with your hands. First inward, circling the hands toward each other 5 to 6 times, and then reverse directions and repeat the circles 5 to 6 times, relaxing your head and neck, allowing most of your weight to rest on the wall. When you have finished this relaxing release, initiate the movement with the abdominals and roll up against the wall bone by bone until you come to standing in perfect posture.

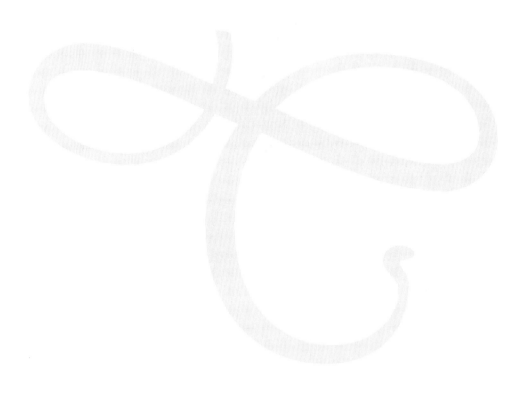

INSIGHT

Allow your body to give in (or give over) completely to the wall behind you so that you feel your body relax entirely. As you begin to round forward, imagine that you are connected to the wall behind you via a heavy spring that is attached to your spine. The spring supports your every move and helps you to roll down slowly and deliberately into the arm circle section. As you roll down into the circle section, you should feel a sense of control and buoyancy. This carries through to the end of the exercise when you uncurl through the spine, lifting into the starting position. This is a "dessert" exercise, a reward for all of your hard work. It will help to relieve neck and shoulder tension and leave you feeling both relaxed and invigorated. Enjoy it!

A calm, meditative breath that clears the sinuses, balances the sides of the brain, stills the body, and quiets the mind.

1. *Sit cross-legged on the floor and place the back of your left hand on your left knee. With the thumb and index fingers of your left hand touching, allow the middle, ring, and pinky fingers to extend gently over your knee. Hold your right hand out in front of you and fold the index and middle fingers into your palm, leaving your ring and pinky fingers and thumb extended.*

2. *Inhale through your nose and block both nostrils by clamping the pinky and ring fingers onto the left nostril and the thumb onto the right. Hold your breath for a moment and then exhale through the right nostril by releasing the thumb while continuing to hold and block the left nostril.*

3. *After exhaling completely, inhale through the same (right) nostril. Block both nostrils and retain the breath for a 5 or 6 count, then exhale for a 5 or 6 count, this time through the left nostril. Inhale again, left, retain the breath, and exhale right. Inhale right, retain the breath, and exhale left. As you grow more comfortable with this exercise, try to extend the inhalation retention and exhalation from 5 or 6 count to 8 or 9.*

4. *Continue for at least 6 to 8 breath cycles. Can you feel your sinuses beginning to open? Are you beginning to feel relaxed? You are ready for meditation.*

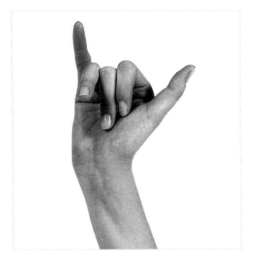

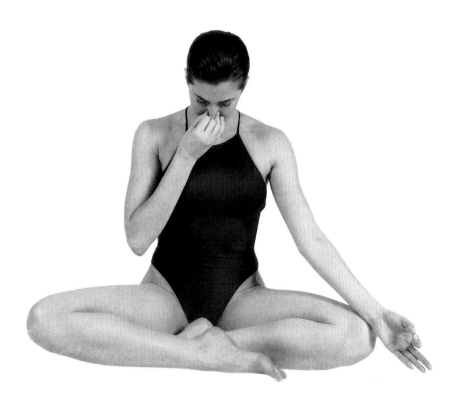

INSIGHT

Truly envision each side of your breathing apparatus when you do alternate nostril breathing. See your inhalations and exhalations as moments for sweeping clean the internal workings of your sinus cavities. As you inhale through the right nostril and close and block both, trust your ability to retain your breath. You will find that if you think this way, you will approach the notion of retention with greater calm and comfort and cultivate greater energy and improved breathing ability as a result.

MEDITATION (YOGA)

Meditation is the hard-earned reward you can look forward to after every exercise session, following the ballet section of the workout. Take a few minutes (preferably 10 minutes initially, and eventually 20) to sit in a comfortable cross-legged position on a lovely cushion or meditation block. Close your eyes, clear your mind, and breathe. The benefits, after the mind and body have been so fully integrated as they are in a workout, are innumerable. Along with proper sleep, diet, and exercise, meditation is a most powerful antidote to the stresses and strains of our everyday lives.

1. *Sit in a comfortable cross-legged position on the floor or in a chair and close your eyes. Inhale and exhale in the ujjayi style (page 38) and then begin alternate nostril breathing (page 232).*

2. *Do several rounds of alternate nostril breathing and then bring the back of your right hand to rest on your right knee. Continue to breathe without effort—just natural, full diaphragmatic breaths. Allow the stomach to expand and release easily.*

3. *Turn your attention and your perceptions inward. Listen to the sounds of your breath. Listen to your heartbeat. Don't allow external sounds to distract you. Energy follows the mind, so if you maintain your focus, your internal energy will gather and you will begin to feel a sense of stillness and calm.*

4. *Focus on the rhythm and the quality of your breath and you will feel lighter and more centered, more peaceful, more grounded.*

5. *Keeping the eyes closed, bring your palms together in front of your heart as a symbol of honor, a way of paying homage to (or of acknowledging) the introspective journey you have just taken.*

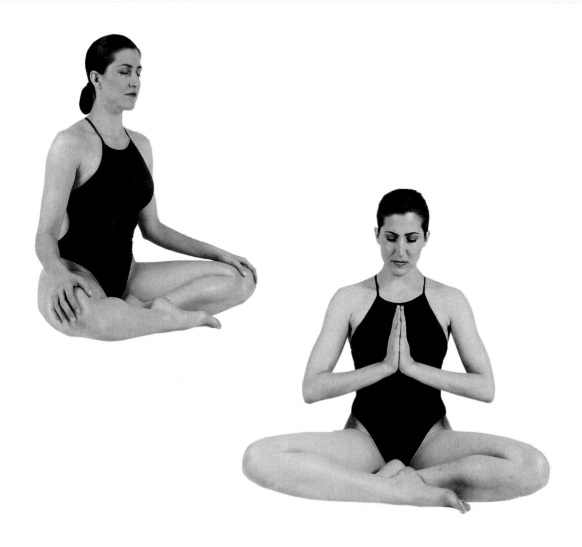

INSIGHT

Don't *try* to meditate. That is the key. Allow your thoughts to wander where they will like an untethered horse, and then gently bring your mind back to the notion of nothingness. For me, nothingness means conjuring a beautiful nature scene, looking at a large, blank, blue-white sky inside my head. Don't chastise yourself for allowing your mind to wander; simply let it go where it wants—when you don't try to tether the horse, he will come to eat out of your hand when you least expect it.

SAVASANA (YOGA)

The very last "pose" you will do, Savasana, is the Corpse Pose, or pose of relaxation in yoga. Relaxes each and every part of the body, encouraging surrender and promoting total peace and well-being. You will do this at the very end of your workout, after meditation.

1. *Lie on the floor and fully extend your body, reaching your arms up overhead and stretching your legs as far away from your center as possible.*

2. *Find a place of complete comfort for every part of your body and allow it to surrender its weight completely into the floor. Truly feel as though the floor were holding your body up.*

3. *Make sure you find a comfortable position for your head and that the curve of your neck naturally establishes itself against the floor. Do the same in regard to your lower back. Make sure you have established your natural lumbar curve against the floor.*

4. *Allow your legs to fall open, and bring your arms down by your sides with the palms facing the ceiling.*

5. *Take several deep and complete breaths, allowing the diaphragm to fill with air and empty without any effort. Let your body take over, and then as you travel through each part of your body, starting with the crown of your head, breathe into each part and then let it go.*

6. *Travel through your body, starting at the crown of your head until you reach your toes and the soles of your feet.*

INSIGHT

This is sure to become a favorite—it's definitely one of mine, something I look forward to after a hard workout. Think flotation tank, think levitation. Allow your entire body to surrender to the floor. Remember, it will support you in every sense, from your head to your feet, your heart, your mind, your soul—no matter what your state of mind.

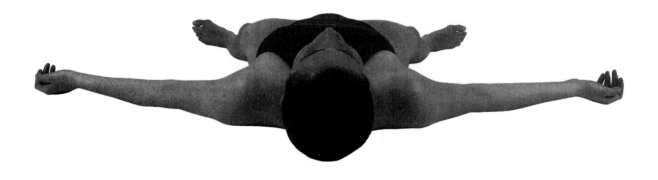

SAVASANA

6

"ON THE FLY": SPORTS SPECIFICS AND TIME-SAVERS

Keep the faculty of effort alive in you by a little gratuitous exercise

every day. That is, be systematically ascetic or heroic in little

unnecessary points, do every day or two something for

no other reason than that you would rather not do it,

so that when the hour of dire need draws nigh,

it may find you not unnerved and untrained

to stand the test.

—William James

SIDE FROM BEING an unparalleled workout on its own, the Method can provide the most significant and all-encompassing platform for cross-training and the most effective, well-rounded foundation for *any* sport or leisure activity, any time, any place—bar none! It helps the body learn to adopt a balanced facility in every plane of movement and develops symmetrical strength through every range of motion. As a result, your ability—your overall stamina and sheer prowess—increases as you develop greater awareness of your body and its subtleties.

Investing your time in this well-balanced workout will unquestionably give you the leading edge in every competition, the advantage in every aspect of your every pursuit. While others will be preoccupied with their body's limitations or concerned about injuring or overextending themselves, *your* body will be functioning at an optimal level, *your* muscles working at peak efficiency, *you* will be free to move through every range of motion, free to move through every endeavor, any sport or physical activity, with the extra measure of strength and energy and confidence that will enable you to dominate your game.

Golfers will enjoy greater torque and longer drives, overall precision and balance; ice-skaters, higher jumps and smoother landings, faster turns and easier transitions. Football players, greater distance on kickoffs and greater agility in plays, greater flexibility and stamina; tennis players will appreciate acing more serves, increased strength and flexibility at the net . . . and the list goes on.

Whether your chosen sport is golf, tennis, swimming, downhill or cross-country skiing, ice-skating, Rollerblading, soccer, basketball, football, ballroom dancing, martial arts, gymnastics, diving, sailing, windsurfing, hiking, mountaineering, cycling, baseball, rowing, fly-fishing, horseback riding (have I left anyone out?)—whether you are a professional football player or a late-blooming ballerina, whatever your leisure activity or athletic pursuit, the Method will revolutionize the way you approach your passion and will enhance it in every way. Regardless of the specific sport, you will experience increased power of the center, which means benefit both on the sheerly physical and on the mental and emotional planes. The positive "domino theory" takes effect. When you experience increased strength in your center, your emotional life becomes more sound, broadening your potential for greater confidence, increased belief in yourself, and greater happiness!

I have selected nine widely practiced sports or physical activities—golf, tennis, skiing, ice- and roller-skating, cycling, running and walking, basketball, swimming, and climbing—and have accompanied each with an appropriate workout and a brief description of the ways in which the Method Workout will improve and enhance key aspects of that particular sport. The kapalabhati and alternate nostril breathing segments are essential to all of these endeavors. Not only will they enable you to warm up, preparing your body for each activity, but they will calm you and balance the mind and body, enhancing concentration and focus. With a clear mind and a balanced body you will be free to follow your sport.

When you aim for perfection, you discover it's a moving target.

—George Fisher

GOLF

Precision, balance, control, torque, distance, are just a few of the important notions that come to mind when you think of golf. You can generate greater torque when you rotate your upper body against your lower body; by virtue of strengthening the core muscles and augmenting balance, you can enhance the power of your swing and increase driving distance, precision, and control. In golf the strength of a properly executed swing begins with your center and rotates your upper body against your lower body, giving your shots the power they need. Because the Method focuses on building the abdominal core, you have immediate access to more power at all times. Not only will your drives gain greater distance and accuracy, but because of the Method breathing techniques, you will be able to maintain a higher level of concentration and control throughout your game. Your flexibility in your shoulders and upper back will increase by virtue of the opening stretches you'll do. You'll feel stronger in your center and be better able to maintain good posture all day, especially on the links.

Here is a series that emphasizes strengthening the muscles of the torso to increase torque and range in the core body and to refine standing posture for improved balance, symmetry, and accuracy. In the workout, concentrate on those exercises that will enhance the body's torque, those exercises that strengthen the internal and external obliques, such as the Crisscross, and those that strengthen the rectus abdominus and other primary abdominal muscles, such as the Hundred through the Double-Leg Lower Lift. In addition, to enhance your core flexibility, spend more time on exercises like the Spine Twist and the Saw.

Kapalabhati Breathing	90
Head and Body Roll	96
The Hundred	98
Pre-Roll-Up	100
Roll-Up	102
Rolling Like a Ball	106
Single-Leg Pull	108
Double-Leg Stretch	110
Scissors	112
Double-Leg Lower Lift	114
Crisscross	116
Spine Stretch Forward	120

THE
GOLF
WORKOUT

Saw	128
Pillow	130
Cat-Cow Combination	132
Active Cat with Yoga Press	136
Cobra	138
Double-Leg Kick	142
Down Dog	150
Spine Twist	158
Side Series	162
Pendulum	164
Inner Thigh Crossover	170
Teaser Series	178
Single-Bent-Leg Teaser	178
Classic Teaser	180
Swimming	184
Seal	186
Sun Salutation	194
Plié Series	204
Tendu en Croix	208
Standing Sculpting Series	214
Alternate Nostril Breathing	232
Meditation	234
Savasana	236

TENNIS

In tennis and other racquet sports, hand-eye coordination is key. So, too, is the power and accuracy of your stroke. But your swing is only as powerful as the source that initiates and fuels it: the power of your core. You will begin to notice, if you haven't already, that the power of all sports (and all movements in life) comes from your center. The strength in your legs and in your arms is equally as important as speed and agility. Imagine what occurs when you are able to successfully balance the strength in both sides of your body! The tennis workout features exercises that strengthen the core but also exercises that focus on increasing strength in the legs to protect against injury during lunges and short stops during net play, and back and upper-body strengtheners for increased range of motion in serves and backhand shots. Focus on upper-body strengtheners such as the Plank with Battements (which strengthens the lower body as well) and the Standing Sculpting Series, and for lower-body strength, the Pelvic Lift with Leg Extension; in the yoga series the Incline Plank, Sun Salutation, Sun Salutation Warrior II, and Hip Flexor Series with Lunges; and the Plié Series in the dance section, to name only a few.

THE TENNIS WORKOUT

Kapalabhati Breathing	90
Pull-Down	94
Head and Body Roll	96
The Hundred	98
Pre-Roll-Up	100
Roll-Up	102
Rolling Like a Ball	106
Single-Leg Pull	108
Double-Leg Stretch	110
Scissors	112
Double-Leg Lower Lift	114
Crisscross	116
Pelvic Lift with Leg Extension	118
Spine Stretch Forward	120
Corkscrew	126
Saw	128
Cat-Cow Combination	132
Active Moving Cat	134
Active Cat with Yoga Press	136
Cobra	138
Single-Leg Kick	140
Double-Leg Kick	142
Flat Yoga Press	146
Plank with Battements	148
Down Dog	150
Spine Twist	158
Side Series	162
Teaser Series	178
Single-Bent-Leg Teaser	178
Classic Teaser	180

Swimming	184
Seal	186
Incline Plank	192
Sun Salutation	194
Hip Flexor Series with Lunges	200
Sun Salutation Warrior II	202
Plié Series	204
Tendu en Croix	208
Dégagé	210
Fondu	212
Standing Sculpting Series	214
Alternate Nostril Breathing	232
Meditation	234
Savasana	236

SKIING AND SKATING

It isn't that I find danger ennobling, or that I require cheap excitation to cure the dullness of routine; but I do like the moment central to danger and to some sports, when you become so thoroughly concerned with acting deftly, in order to be safe, that only reaction is possible, not analysis. You shed the centuries and feel creatural. Of course, you do have to scan, assess, and make constant minute decisions. But there is nothing like thinking in the usual, methodical way. What takes its place is more akin to an informed instinct. For a pensive person, to be fully alert but free of thought is a form of ecstasy. . . . There is also a state when perception doesn't work, consciousness vanishes like the gorgeous fever it is, and you feel free of all mind-body constraints, suddenly so free of them you don't perceive yourself as being free, but vigilant, a seeing eye without judgment, history or emotion. It's that shudder out of time, the central moment in so many sports, that one often feels, and perhaps becomes addicted to, while doing something dangerous.

—Diane Ackerman

In sports such as skiing (cross-country, downhill, or waterskiing) and skating (on wheels or on ice), integral to your performance is the strength in the legs as well as an overall balance and symmetry, which again emanates from the core, so that as you glide over your chosen surface, be it water, ice, or snow, you are in command of your body and will feel in complete harmony with the surfaces nature provides.

The exercises for skiing and skating emphasize flexibility in the legs and back (for injury prevention) and range of motion in the hamstrings and lower back (strengthening the adductors, or inner thigh muscles, which need to counterbalance the work of the abductors, or outer thighs). Concentrate on the Inner Thigh Crossover in the Side Series for these.

You should also focus on lower-body and core-strengthening exercises (which will also slim and lengthen the muscle bodies) like the Pelvic Lift with Leg Extension, Single-Leg Kick, Double-Leg Kick, Sun Salutation Warrior II, Hip Flexor Series with Lunges, pliés—tendus, dégagés, fondu—and of course the classic Pilates core exercises, starting with the Hundred. For flexibility, each time you do forward bending (whether it be in the actual Seated Forward Bend or in the "swan dive" portion of the Sun Salutation), take your time and breathe through the stretch and you will steadily increase your flexibility along with your core strength.

Kapalabhati Breathing	90
Roll-Down	92
Pull-Down	94
Head and Body Roll	96
The Hundred	98
Pre-Roll-Up	100
Roll-Up	102
Rolling Like a Ball	106
Single-Leg Pull	108
Double-Leg Stretch	110
Scissors	112
Double-Leg Lower Lift	114
Crisscross	116
Pelvic Lift with Leg Extension	118
Spine Stretch Forward	120
Open-Leg Rocker	122
Corkscrew	126
Saw	128
Cat-Cow Combination	132
Active Moving Cat	134
Active Cat with Yoga Press	136
Cobra	138
Single-Leg Kick	140
Double-Leg Kick	142
Flat Yoga Press	146
Plank with Battements	148
Down Dog Nose to Knee	152
Neck Pull	154
Rollover	156
Spine Twist	158
Seated Forward Bend	160
Side Series	162
Teaser Series	178
Single-Bent-Leg Teaser	178
Classic Teaser	180

THE SKIING AND SKATING WORKOUT

THE SKIING AND SKATING WORKOUT

Swimming	184
Sun Salutation	194
Hip Flexor Series with Lunges	200
Sun Salutation Warrior II	202
Plié Series	204
Tendu en Croix	208
Dégagé	210
Fondu	212
Standing Sculpting Series	214
Alternate Nostril Breathing	232
Meditation	234
Savasana	236

CYCLING

In cycling, because of the rounded, crouched position one must assume, most important are strength and flexibility for the legs, enhanced power in the core for stabilization and the initiation of pedaling, and counterstretching for the spine. In a sport like cycling, it is not only important to stretch and strengthen the legs for pedaling over all types of terrain; equally necessary are strength and range of motion in opposition to or as a countermeasure for the constantly held positions and repetitive movements that cycling requires.

To strengthen and condition the legs, these are the exercises you should spend more time on: Pelvic Lift with Leg Extension, Single-Leg Kick, Double-Leg Kick, Side Series, Swimming, Sun Salutation Warrior II, Hip Flexor Series with Lunges, pliés—tendus, dégagés, fondu. And to open the chest and shoulders and release tension in the spine, these exercises are unbeatable: Spine Twist, Spine Stretch Forward, Cat-Cow Combination, Cobra, Single-Leg Kick, and Double-Leg Kick.

Kapalabhati Breathing	90
Roll-Down	92
Pull-Down	94
Head and Body Roll	96
The Hundred	98
Pre–Roll-Up	100
Roll-Up	102
Leg Circles	104
Rolling Like a Ball	106
Single-Leg Pull	108
Double-Leg Stretch	110
Scissors	112
Double-Leg Lower Lift	114
Crisscross	116
Pelvic Lift with Leg Extension	118
Spine Stretch Forward	120
Open-Leg Rocker	122
Corkscrew	126
Saw	128
Cat-Cow Combination	132
Active Moving Cat	134
Cobra	138
Single-Leg Kick	140
Double-Leg Kick	142
Plank with Battements	148
Down Dog Nose to Knee	152
Neck Pull	154
Rollover	156
Spine Twist	158
Seated Forward Bend	160
Side Series	162
Teaser Series	178
Single-Bent-Leg Teaser	178
Classic Teaser	180
Swimming	184
Sun Salutation	194
Hip Flexor Series with Lunges	200
Sun Salutation Warrior II	202

THE CYCLING WORKOUT

Plié Series		204
Tendu en Croix		208
Dégagé		210
Fondu		212
Standing Sculpting Series		214
Alternate Nostril Breathing		232
Meditation		234
Savasana		236

RUNNING AND WALKING

What are the keys to injury prevention that will add longevity to your running or walking career? Strength in the legs, stamina, endurance, focus? What about flexibility and the strength in your core? Well, here's a workout for all you runners and walkers out there—guaranteed to ease some of the impact on your lower body and on your back. Special attention will be given to increasing flexibility and core strength.

Make sure you concentrate and really breathe, even through the portions of the exercises that emphasize stretching (like the Seated Forward Bend and the Roll-Up). If you take your time with the stretches and extend the length of time during which you hold them, you will benefit tremendously, and although walking has less impact on the lower body and back than running, the same workout is effective for both running and walking.

The exercises I have selected are also those that will strengthen, slim, and lengthen the muscles of the legs, creating a greater ratio of balance between the hamstrings and the quadriceps (which do a great deal of the work in running, often leading to tight, underutilized hamstrings).

The Running Workout

Roll-Down, Roll-Up, the Pilates core exercises, beginning with the Hundred (lingering on any forward-bending stretches you encounter and emphasizing the Scissors to increase hamstring flexibility), Pelvic Lift with

Leg Extension, Spine Stretch Forward, Open-Leg Rocker (especially great for increasing the range of motion in your hamstrings), Corkscrew, Saw, Plank with Battements, Down Dog Nose to Knee, Neck Pull (remember to stretch as deeply as possible on the forward-bending portion of this and all similar exercises), Rollover (this will be especially challenging at first because of the tightness in your hamstring insertion, the place where the hamstrings join into the gluteals, which are connected to the lower back; stick with this one—it is very effective in opening the hamstring-back connection and will keep your back resilient, healthy, and strong), Spine Twist, Seated Forward Bend, Teaser Series, Sun Salutation, Hip Flexor Series with Lunges, and the Ballet Series through dégagé.

Kapalabhati Breathing	90
Roll-Down	92
Pull-Down	94
Head and Body Roll	96
The Hundred	98
Pre-Roll-Up	100
Roll-Up	102
Rolling Like a Ball	106
Single-Leg Pull	108
Double-Leg Stretch	110
Scissors	112
Double-Leg Lower Lift	114
Crisscross	116
Pelvic Lift with Leg Extension	118
Spine Stretch Forward	120
Open-Leg Rocker	122
Corkscrew	126
Saw	128
Cat-Cow Combination	132
Active Moving Cat	134
Active Cat with Yoga Press	136
Cobra	138
Single-Leg Kick	140
Double-Leg Kick	142
Flat Yoga Press	146

THE RUNNING
AND
WALKING
WORKOUT

THE RUNNING AND WALKING WORKOUT	
Plank with Battements	142
Down Dog Nose to Knee	152
Neck Pull	154
Rollover	156
Spine Twist	158
Seated Forward Bend	160
Side Series	162
Teaser Series	178
Single-Bent-Leg Teaser	178
Classic Teaser	180
Swimming	184
Sun Salutation	194
Hip Flexor Series with Lunges	200
Sun Salutation Warrior II	202
Plié Series	204
Tendu en Croix	208
Dégagé	210
Fondu	212
Standing Sculpting Series	214
Alternate Nostril Breathing	232
Meditation	234
Savasana	236

BASKETBALL

The dodges, the passes, the short stops, the big jumps and leaps to the basket, the dancing around your opponent! You really need to be in complete control of your torso as it twists and turns in an effort to grab the ball away from the other side, maneuver it down the court, and keep it once you've grabbed it. Your legs have to be strong and flexible to jump high and make those slam dunks, your upper body just as strong and supple, and your coordination, speed, and agility in top form. In this workout, you will concentrate primarily on building your abdominal core and hand-eye coordination (Single-Leg Pull and Double-Leg Kick on the stomach are two good ones for this drill), and then work outward, building balanced strength in your arms and legs.

Kapalabhati Breathing	90
Roll-Down	92
Pull-Down	94
Head and Body Roll	96
The Hundred	98
Pre-Roll-Up	100
Roll-Up	102
Rolling Like a Ball	106
Single-Leg Pull	108
Double-Leg Stretch	110
Scissors	112
Double-Leg Lower Lift	114
Crisscross	116
Pelvic Lift with Leg Extension	118
Spine Stretch Forward	120
Open-Leg Rocker	122
Corkscrew	126
Saw	128
Cat-Cow Combination	132
Active Moving Cat	134
Active Cat with Yoga Press	136
Cobra	138
Single-Leg Kick	140
Double-Leg Kick	142
Flat Yoga Press	146
Plank with Battements	148
Down Dog Nose to Knee	152
Neck Pull	154
Rollover	156
Spine Twist	158
Seated Forward Bend	160
Side Series	162
Teaser Series	178
Single-Bent-Leg Teaser	178
Classic Teaser	180
Swimming	184
Sun Salutation	194
Hip Flexor Series with Lunges	200
Sun Salutation Warrior II	202

THE
BASKETBALL
WORKOUT

THE
BASKETBALL
WORKOUT

Plié Series	204
Tendu en Croix	208
Dégagé	210
Fondu	212
Standing Sculpting Series	214
Alternate Nostril Breathing	232
Meditation	234
Savasana	236

SWIMMING

I want to stay as close to the edge as I can without going over. Out on the edge you see all kinds of things you can't see from the center.
—Kurt Vonnegut

Swimming provides a total body workout that is in many ways similar to the integrative training inherent in the Method. The upper and lower body develop in beautiful proportion and the strength in the core body is usually quite strong as compared with the level of core strength produced in other sports. In order to propel the body forward and backward underwater with speed and economy of movement, the body's motion initiates from the center and moves outward, immediately engaging arms and legs, contributing to graceful and powerful locomotion. The body moves against a substantial amount of resistance as it moves through the water, and in this way swimming shares yet another dimension in common with the exercises of the Method. All the exercises in the Method require that you work with your own self-imposed isometric resistance to sculpt long, lean, strong, and flexible muscles.

In swimming, to increase speed and efficiency of movement, a fully balanced workout is in order. I recommend that you concentrate on upper-body exercises that both strengthen and open the chest and shoulders (similar to the list for cyclists, including those that provide a counter-stretch), exercises that increase the power of your center (the full Pilates core exercises), and of course, those exercises that strengthen the legs. Additionally, because of the more complicated and synergistic movement patterns that are characteristic of strokes like the butterfly and the backstroke, I suggest you try your hand at perfecting the more advanced exercises that involve a greater number of elements that enhance upper-body and lower-body strength and flexibility simultaneously, such as the Plank with Battements, Rollover, the Side Series (especially Ronde de Jambe and Hot Potato), Jackknife, Boomerang, and some of the more straightforward of the exercises—and of course, Swimming.

Kapalabhati Breathing	90
Roll-Down	92
Pull-Down	94
Head and Body Roll	96
The Hundred	98
Pre–Roll-Up	100
Roll-Up	102
Rolling Like a Ball	106
Single-Leg Pull	108
Double-Leg Stretch	110
Scissors	112
Double-Leg Lower Lift	114
Crisscross	116
Pelvic Lift with Leg Extension	118
Spine Stretch Forward	120
Open-Leg Rocker	122
Corkscrew	126
Saw	128
Cat-Cow Combination	132
Active Moving Cat	134
Active Cat with Yoga Press	136
Cobra	138
Single-Leg Kick	140
Double-Leg Kick	142
Flat Yoga Press	146
Plank with Battements	148
Down Dog Nose to Knee	152
Neck Pull	154
Rollover	156
Spine Twist	158
Seated Forward Bend	160
Side Series	162

THE SWIMMING WORKOUT

THE SWIMMING WORKOUT

Jackknife	176
Teaser Series	178
Swimming	184
Boomerang	188
Incline Plank	192
Sun Salutation	194
Hip Flexor Series with Lunges	200
Sun Salutation Warrior II	202
Plié Series	204
Tendu en Croix	208
Dégagé	210
Fondu	212
Standing Sculpting Series	214
Alternate Nostril Breathing	232
Meditation	234
Savasana	236

CLIMBING

We stand on the brink of a precipice. We peer into the abyss—we grow sick and dizzy. Our first impulse is to shrink from the danger. Unaccountably we remain.
—Edgar Allan Poe

Climbing, a sport that requires total concentration and focus, sheer determination, great courage, and a penchant for pure risk, also requires a total balanced strength in core, arms, and legs. Balance and tenacity, elasticity and strength in all aspects, are prerequisites for serious climbers. In order to balance on narrow passes high above menacing crevasses, to pull your entire body weight from precarious perch to precarious perch and maneuver your hands and feet with agility and control, you must hone substantial core strength and skill. I have created a workout that underscores the power of your center and balanced strength in your upper body and lower body, along with exercises that demand precision and balance (Rolling Like a Ball, Open-Leg Rocker, Teaser Series, Side Series) and those that challenge your ability to risk and ask you to venture into the more complicated, multilayer aspects of the exercises, including the Rollover, Jackknife, and Boomerang, among others. Make sure that you spend extra time on the rocking and rolling exercises, such as Rolling Like a Ball and the Open-Leg Rocker. Try to establish your balance immediately and apply yourself to maintaining your balance with your breath, your focus, and your core.

Kapalabhati Breathing	90
Pull-Down	94
Head and Body Roll	96
The Hundred	98
Pre-Roll-Up	100
Roll-Up	102
Rolling Like a Ball	106
Single-Leg Pull	108
Double-Leg Stretch	110
Scissors	112
Double-Leg Lower Lift	114
Crisscross	116
Pelvic Lift with Leg Extension	118
Spine Stretch Forward	120
Open-Leg Rocker	122
Corkscrew	126
Saw	128
Cat-Cow Combination	132
Active Moving Cat	134
Active Cat with Yoga Press	136
Cobra	138
Single-Leg Kick	140
Double-Leg Kick	142
Flat Yoga Press	146
Plank with Battements	148
Down Dog Nose to Knee	152
Neck Pull	154
Rollover	156
Spine Twist	158
Seated Forward Bend	160
Side Series	162
Jackknife	176
Teaser Series	178
Swimming	184
Boomerang	188
Incline Plank	192

THE CLIMBING WORKOUT

THE CLIMBING WORKOUT

Sun Salutation	194
Hip Flexor Series with Lunges	200
Sun Salutation Warrior II	202
Plié Series	204
Tendu en Croix	208
Dégagé	210
Fondu	212
Standing Sculpting Series	214
Alternate Nostril Breathing	232
Meditation	234
Savasana	236

ON THE FLY . . . THE TIME-SAVERS

Here are two timesaving twenty-minute programs I call On the Fly. Each is a complete body workout designed for those enthusiasts for whom time is a luxury, who would want to follow the complete Method Workout but who, because of time constraints, require an abbreviated version. The two total-body workout combinations can be done before or after work, as a supplement to your "sporting hour," in a hotel room, or in your own living room. You will find them to be surprisingly complete. Although they don't offer the entire menu, you can still move through every range of motion and use all the muscles you would in the more complete workouts of levels 1, 2, and 3.

Each of the following workouts contains key elements for the entire body on your respective level and takes a total of twenty minutes from beginning to end. Enjoy!

WORKOUT I (Beginner)

Kapalabhati Breathing	90
Roll-Down	92
Head and Body Roll	96
The Hundred	98
Pre–Roll-Up	100
Roll-Up	102
Rolling Like a Ball	106

Single-Leg Pull   108
Scissors   112
Crisscross   116
Pelvic Lift with Leg Extension   118
Spine Stretch Forward   120
Open-Leg Rocker (Preparation)   122
Saw   128
Pillow   130
Cat-Cow Combination   132
Cobra   138
Single-Leg Kick   140
Active Moving Cat   134
Down Dog   150
Seated Forward Bend   160
Side Series   162
    Pendulum   164
    Toss-Up   166
Teaser Series   178
    Single-Bent-Leg Teaser   178
    Classic Teaser   180
Swimming   184
Seal   186
Sun Salutation   194
Plié Series   204
    First Position   204
    Second Position   206
    Tendu en Croix   208
    Dégagé   210
    Fondu   212
Standing Sculpting Series   214
90-Degree Front Press Forward   214
Strongman   216
Side Bend   218
Alternate Nostril Breathing   232
Meditation   234
Savasana   236

WORKOUT I
(Beginner)

WORKOUT II
(Intermediate and Advanced)

Kapalabhati Breathing	90
Pull-Down	92
Head and Body Roll	96
The Hundred	98
Roll-Up	102
Leg Circles	104
Rolling Like a Ball	106
Single-Leg Pull	108
Double-Leg Stretch	110
Scissors	112
Double-Leg Lower Lift	114
Crisscross	116
Pelvic Lift with Leg Extension	118
Spine Stretch Forward	120
Open-Leg Rocker	122
Corkscrew	126
Saw	128
Active Cat with Yoga Press	136
Single-Leg Kick	140
Double-Leg Kick	142
Flat Yoga Press	146
Plank with Battements	148
Down Dog Nose to Knee	152
Neck Pull	154
Rollover	156
Spine Twist	158
Seated Forward Bend	160
Side Series	162
Pendulum	164
Toss-Up	166
Bicycle	168
Inner Thigh Crossover	170
Ronde de Jambe	172
Hot Potato	174
Teaser Series	178
Classic Teaser	180
Arms-to-Ears Teaser	182
Swimming	184

Seal	186
Incline Plank	192
Hip Flexor Series with Lunges	200
Sun Salutation Warrior II	202
Plié Series	204
First Position	204
Second Position	206
Tendu en Croix	208
Dégagé	210
Fondu	212
Standing Sculpting Series	214
90-Degrees Front Press	214
Strongman	216
Side Bend	218
Chest Expansion	220
Boxing	222
Alternate Nostril Breathing	232
Meditation	234
Savasana	236

WORKOUT II
(Intermediate
and
Advanced)

TAKING IT WITH YOU: THE METHOD FOR LIFE!

Our deepest fear is not that we are inadequate. Our deepest fear is that we are powerful beyond measure. It is our light, not our darkness, that most frightens us. We ask ourselves,"Who am I to be brilliant, gorgeous, talented, fabulous?" Actually, who are you not to be?

—Nelson Mandela

HIS IS NOT just a book about exercise but a book about how to make exercise a part of your life. My goal is for you to enjoy yourself in the realm of fitness, to use Jennifer Kries' Pilates Plus Method as a guide and vehicle for your own personal expansion and transformation.

The Method is not just a workout but a philosophy, one that will inspire you to be the best that you can be. It will grow with you for the rest of your life and deepen the way you experience your own value. Once you see how invigorated you feel, how wonderful you look, how every activity and every aspect of your life improves, the Method Workout will become as essential to you as eating or breathing. It is easy and accessible, a workout that will "stick," where others have failed or fallen by the wayside, the inspiration that will lead you to say "Yes!"

When you start the Method program, know that it will take some time to develop your body and the capacity to endure the physical and mental demands placed upon it. When obstacles arise, don't fight them or become discouraged; accept and acknowledge them. Look upon them as an opportunity to assess your abilities and to learn as you grow stronger. With patience and determination, you will find resolution and progress. Exercise should not be thought of as punishment but as a way to lighten the load, to take a minivacation from daily life that will leave you rejuvenated when you return. As you learn to feel, to know exactly what your body is doing, exercise becomes more pleasant. Concentrating over a period of time on centering, control, precision, flowing motion, and breathing results in the growth of a powerful sense of well-being and confidence. Learning, growth, and integration—like the changes in the shape of your body—are brought about by the activity itself without conscious stress on the goals.

The exercises in this book will change the shape of your body if done faithfully and consistently. As you come to discover a new freedom in your body, your mind and soul will follow. The effects are dramatic and immediate. After just two or three sessions, you will see and feel the results.

Despite the alternative-health and fitness revolution that we have witnessed over the past decade, which erupted in reaction to the business push to achieve and amass more and more and the "no pain, no gain" mentality, people are only now beginning to discover that changing the shape of the body and personal transformation are subtle processes that require inspiration, determination, commitment, and patience. With this workout you will come to discover that the two are inextricably linked. We have all had (at one time or another) the unfortunate experience of feeling that we were at the mercy of our bodies when they did not perform as we would have liked, but this seemingly unfortunate experience is in fact the very thing that initiates self-discovery.

The pleasure and satisfaction of movement for its own sake are available to every person. The nature of the Method is such that it inspires everyone to become more goal oriented because of the immediate and abundant rewards. The beauty of the Method lies in the paradox that the work grows easier and more challenging at the same time. Every workout cumulatively increases your strength and flexibility, inspiring you to reach higher and higher. Your previously untapped ability and reserves will unleash focus and concentration, will and desire. You refine the work; perfect every movement, every exercise; and continually raise the bar.

As you grow, so does your confidence, and your body's transformation is mirrored even more profoundly by that of your mind. Deep wells of creativity and thought may be tapped and harnessed, and you learn to value and appreciate growth through process for the very first time. The timeless principles of the Method, this awesome blend of Eastern philosophy and Western athleticism, a never-ending circle of learning, growth, and integration, will bring new balance and harmony into your life and reveal to you who you truly are.

The quest to find your own best self is a very personal and hopeful one. The Method Workout can be the catalyst for your discoveries and help you to access a personal freedom you never would have dreamed possible. A more physical life can encourage you to confront inner feelings and concerns like courage, perseverance, or self-doubt—personal growth far more valuable than any exercise or skill by itself. The sheer elation you experience when you reach the top of a mountain that you never thought you could climb is the same deep soulful connection to life you will feel as you surpass all of your own preconceived limitations and ideas.

Convincing your body to let go of old habits, even those that are obsolete, is no easy task. The body likes what it already knows and is extraordinarily faithful to familiar pathways and patterns. Practice and repetition, dedication and devotion, are all required. It also takes a leap of faith before you can be persuaded (or persuade yourself!) to set out on a different, albeit better, path and begin to move on. But when you are physically stimulated and your mind is directed toward the task at hand, pathways are opened to your inner emotional life, to the real self as well as to the deep centers of creativity and thought. You gain wisdom by going the way of nature instead of opposing it egotistically. Personal power is developed when you cease to be self-critical and merely accept the true natural self. When you are able to accept who you are for all of your strengths in spite of your weakness, you will discover a total strength and peace never known before. Your ultimate power is achieved when you don't seek power at all.

Release yourself from old and outmoded ways of thinking. You *can* learn to reeducate and retrain your body and mind. When you cultivate strength with precision and determination, when you practice the

Method Workout faithfully and consistently, not only will every muscle in your body feel stretched, conditioned, and massaged, but you will look upon every challenge as an opportunity, and instead of becoming depleted or exhausted as you normally would after exercise, you will feel omnipotent, invigorated, energized—whole!

That's why the Method is so exciting! At the close of a forty-five-minute workout the session does not come to an end. Whatever you have learned in any given segment, whether it is a new way to focus your breath or a technique to lengthen and strengthen a muscle, the difference between effortless effort and pushing or how to use a loosely pointed foot, you get to take it all with you. Your ability to multitask expands because everything in the workout provides the body and the brain with a constant subtle drill of your autosensory systems, your coordination skills; the right and left brain are both exercised equally. A profound internal and external transformation takes place—and you have made it happen!

This book is a starting point: an inspiration, promoting economy of movement, focus, a reshaping of lifestyle. It is a portable system for a portable world. Even in our mobile society, where travel is a way of life, no one has created a gym you can take with you as you would your cellular phone or your laptop computer. Until now. As your portable gym, once the Method becomes a part of your life, you will have a foundation for everything else you do, a platform for cross-training, a resource, a tool, a companion. You take it with you wherever you go and use what you have learned every minute of every day as you discover new ways to walk, talk, reach, bend, garden, think, make love, run, work, play.

Every activity in your life, from gardening to sex, will become more pleasurable and more unburdening when your body is so fit and so capable that you are able to be in the moment. Your mind and spirit will be set free as physical activity becomes a way for you to be at peace and at one with yourself. Every intimate occasion becomes more immediate, more sensual, when you are proud of yourself and your body and at liberty to open yourself to another.

I have intended my book, *Jennifer Kries' Pilates Plus Method*, not as a substitute for the Pilates, yoga, or dance class you may currently be engaged in but rather as an enlightening supplement. I have sprinkled it liberally with many of my secrets and insights and much of my hard-won knowledge of little-known and technical components gained from my experience as an apprentice with three of Joseph Pilates' disciples, as a professional dancer, and from years of yoga study and practice. I hope you have felt my presence and my words of encouragement.

In the end, however, it is up to you. The greater the investment of *your* time in exercise, *your* patience, *your* diligence and mastery, and the more you connect the power of the mind with that of the body, the more your spirit has cause to rejoice, the more ease and facility you will experience, the more harmony and gratification you will bring into your life. This is not just a workout, it is a philosophy. It is a state of mind, a state of being. It is the ultimate fitness for body, mind, and spirit. It can help you transform your life. And it will inspire you to be the very best you can be.

And, if you should individually achieve calmness and harmony in your own person, you may depend upon it that a wave of imitation will spread from you, as surely as the circles spread outward when a stone is dropped into a lake.

—William James

ASSESSMENT

The following form can be used to clarify why you are embarking on your Pilates Plus Method journey and will serve as an outline before you begin. After completing the assessment, read through it as if you were the teacher collecting vital information about a new student. Then take a moment to reflect on this before you enter into a new realm where the body, mind, and spirit become one. If you are interested in a personal consultation, and you would like me to answer questions regarding this evaluation, send the completed form and enclose a check or money order for $35 to Jennifer Kries, The Balanced Body Center, 232 Mercer Street, New York, NY 10012.

Use what talents you possess—the woods would be very silent if no birds sang there except those that sang best.
—Henry Van Dyke

WHO ARE YOU?

Name _____

Address _____

E-mail address _____

Male or female _____

Age _____

Height _____

Weight _____

Profession _____

WHAT IS YOUR BODY TYPE?

Body types: Ectomorph (fine boned with a slight build) Mesomorph (medium boned with a muscular, athletic physique) Endomorph (large boned with a broad build)

Note: You can be a combination of two categories. Where do you tend to carry your extra weight? Would you describe yourself as having a pear shape? An hourglass shape?

Try to describe your body type here: _____

_____

_____

If you could change anything about your body, what would it be? _____

_____

_____

If you could brag about any part of your body, what would it be? _____

_____

_____

TELL ME ABOUT YOUR EXERCISE HISTORY

What do you do to stay fit? _____

_____

_____

_____

_____

Describe an actual exercise week, *for real* and ideal. _____

_____

_____

_____

_____

How much time are you able to dedicate to exercise? _____

_____

_____

_____

What are your exercise goals (e.g., greater stamina, abdominal strength, increased flexibility, a smaller backside, slimmer hips)? _____

_____

_____

_____

How much time are you able to dedicate to exercise? _____

_____

_____

_____

INDEX

Page numbers of photographs and illustrations appear in italics.

Abdominal contraction (establishing the navel-to-spine connection), 26, 41–43 (exercise 11)
Abdominal lock (exercise 4), 34–35
Abdominals (muscles: obliques (internal and external), pyramidalis, rectus abdominus, transversus abdominus), 15, 83
  Active Cat with Yoga Press, 136, *137*
  Active Moving Cat, 134, *135*
  Arm Circles, 228, *229*
  Arms-to-Ears Teaser, 182, *183*
  Boomerang, 188, *189*, 190, *191*
  as "centers" or "core muscles," 6, 13, 15
  Classic Teaser, 180, *181*
  contraction of rectus abdominus, 41–43 (exercise 11)
  Corkscrew, 126, *127*
  Crisscross, 116, *117*
  Double-Leg Lower and Lift, 114, *115*
  Double-Leg Stretch, 110, *111*
  Down Dog Nose to Knee, 152, *153*
  Jackknife, 176, *177*
  Neck Pull, 154, *155*
  Open-Leg Rocker, 124, *125*
  Open-Leg Rocker Prep, 122, *123*
  Pillow, 130, *131*

  Pre-Roll-Up, 100, *101*
  quality and quantity with intuitive integration, 49–50 (exercise 14)
  Rolling like a Ball, 106–7, *107*
  Rollover, 156, *157*
  Roll-Up, 102, *103*
  Scissors, 112, *112*
  Seal, 186, *187*
  Single-Bent-Leg Teaser, 178, *179*
  Single-Leg Kick, 140, *141*
  Single-Leg Pull, 108–9, *109*
  spine and, 41
  Spine Twist, 158, *159*
  strength stressed by Method Workout, 1
Ackerman, Diane, 246
Active Cat with Yoga Press, 136, *137*
  basketball workout, 253
  climbing workout, 257
  golf workout, 244
  running and walking workout, 251
  skiing and skating workout, 247
  swimming workout, 255
  tennis workout, 245
Active Moving Cat, 134, *135*
  basketball workout, 253
  climbing workout, 257
  running and walking workout, 251
  skiing and skating workout, 247
  swimming workout, 255
  tennis workout, 245
Acupuncture, 19

African proverb, 95
Alda, Alan, 48
Ali, Muhammad, 266
Alternate nostril breathing, 19, 30
  basketball workout, 253
  climbing workout, 257
  cycling workout, 250
  exercise 10, 40, 232–33, *232–33*
  golf workout, 244
  running and walking workout, 251
  skiing and skating workout, 248
  swimming workout, 255
  tennis workout, 246
  See also Meditation
Anal lock (mula bhanda; exercise 3), 34–35
Arm Circles, 228, *229*
Arms, 83, 84
  Active Cat with Yoga Press, 136, *137*
  Boxing, 222, *223*
  Corkscrew, 126, *127*
  Dégagé, 210, *211*
  First and Second Positions, 204–5, *205*, 206, *207*
  Flat Yoga Press, 146, *147*
  Fondu, 212, *213*
  The Hundred, 98, *99*
  90-degree front press forward, 214–15, *215*
  Rollover, 156, *157*
  Shaving the Head, 224, *224*
  Side Bend, 218, *219*

Strongman, 216, *216–17*
Tendu en Croix, 208, *209*
Arms-to-Ears Teaser, 182, *183*
Assessment form, 271–73

Back (muscles: latissimus dorsi, rhom-
     boids), 15, *84*
  Active Cat with Yoga Press, 136, *137*
  Active Moving Cat, 134, *135*
  Arm Circles, 228, *229*
  Boomerang, 188, 189, 190, *191*
  Boxing, 222, *223*
  Child's Pose, 144, *145*
  Classic Teaser, 180, *181*
  Cobra, 138, *139*
  Corkscrew, 126, *127*
  Double-Leg Kick, 142, *143*
  Double-Leg Stretch, 110, *111*
  Down Dog, 150, *151*
  Down Dog Nose to Knee, 152, *153*
  Head and Body Roll, 96, *97*
  Hug, 226, *227*
  Jackknife, 176, *177*
  latissimus-trapezius connection,
     78–80
  Leg Circles, 104–5, *105*
  Neck Pull, 154, *155*
  90-Degree Front Press Forward,
     214–15, *215*
  Open-Leg Rocker, 124, *125*
  Open-Leg Rocker Prep, 122, *123*
  Plank with Battements, 148, *149*
  Pre-Roll-Up, 100, *101*
  Roll-Down, 92, *93*
  Rollover, 156, *157*
  Roll-Up, 102, *103*
  Saw, 128, *129*
  Seal, 186, *187*
  Shaving the Head, 224, *224*
  Side Bend, 218, *219*
  Single-Leg Kick, 140, *141*
  spinal articulation, 74–78
  Spine Stretch Forward, 120, *121*
  Spine Twist, 158, *159*
  Strongman, 216, *216–17*
  Sun Salutation, 194, *194–95*, 196,
     197, 198, *199*
  Sun Salutation Warrior II, 202, *203*
  Swimming, 184, *185*
Balance
  benefits of equilibrium, 71

Boomerang, 188, 189, 190, *191*
Chest Expansion, 220, *221*
Dégagé, 210, *211*
dominant and weaker sides, 69, 82
First and Second Positions, 204–5,
     205, 206, *207*
Fondu, 212, *213*
Head and Body Roll, 96, *97*
Hip Flexor Series with Lunges, 200,
     201
Incline Plank, 192, *193*
injury prevention and, 69, 82
90-Degree Front Press Forward,
     214–15, *215*
Open-Leg Rocker, 124, *125*
Open-Leg Rocker Prep, 122, *123*
Pelvic Lift with Leg Extension, 118,
     119
Pilates benefits, 16
Pull-Down, 94, *95*
Rolling like a Ball, 106–7, *107*
Seal, 186, *187*
Shaving the Head, 224, *224*
Side Bend, 218, *219*
Strongman, 216, *216–17*
Tendu en Croix, 208, *209*
Basketball, 252
  workout, 253
Bicycle, 168, *169*
Boomerang, 188, *189*, 190, *191*
  climbing workout, 257
  swimming workout, 255
Boxing, 222, *223*
Brain
  spine as neural pathway to, 76
  sympathetic and parasympathetic
     nerves, 29–30
Breathing, 26, 27–40
  abdominal lock, 34–35(exercise 4)
  alternate nostril, 19, 30, 40 (exercise
     10), 232–33, *232–33*
  anal lock (mula bhanda), 34–35
     (exercise 3)
  basic inhalation and exhalation with
     abdominal contraction, 30
  chi (energy) and, 19, 33
  diaphragm and, 28
  exhalation, 32, 36 (exercise 6)
  full inhalation, retention with the
     three locks, and exhalation, 37
     (exercise 7)

as healing force, 19
  inhalation, 30, 32
  kapalabhati, breath of fire, 19, 30,
     39 (exercise 9), 90, *91*
  learning to breathe, 30–31 (exercise
     1)
  muscles involved, 28
  retention, 30, 31, 32, 33
  retention and the three locks, 33–38
  rhythm of, 13, 37–40
  throat lock, 35–36 (exercise 5)
  ujjayi, 19, 30, 38 (exercise 8)
  understanding retention, 33–34
     (exercise 2)
  yoga and, 7, 18–19
Buttocks (muscles: erector spinae,
     quadratus lumborum, gluteus
     maximus), 15, *84*
  Active Moving Cat, 134, *135*
  Bicycle, 168, *169*
  Cobra, 138, *139*
  Dégagé, 210, *211*
  First and Second Positions, 204–5,
     205, 206, *207*
  Fondu, 212, *213*
  Hip Flexor Series with Lunges, 200,
     201
  Hot Potato, 174, *175*
  Inner Thigh Crossover, 170, *171*
  Jackknife, 176, *177*
  Leg Circles, 104–5, *105*
  90-Degree Front Press Forward,
     214–15, *215*
  Pendulum, 164, *165*
  Plank with Battements, 148, *149*
  Pull-Down, 94, *95*
  Ronde de Jambe, 172, *173*
  Shaving the Head, 224, *224*
  Side Bend, 218, *219*
  Single-Leg Kick, 140, *141*
  Spine Stretch Forward, 120, *121*
  Strongman, 216, *216–17*
  Swimming, 184, *185*
  Tendu en Croix, 208, *209*
  Toss-Up, 166, *167*
  turned out position and, 67

Campfire Breathing, or seated prepara-
     tion for the Hundred Breath (Pre-
     exercise No. 6), 73–74
Carnegie, Dale, 61

Cat-Cow Combination, 132, *133*
  basketball workout, 253
  climbing workout, 257
  cycling workout, 249
  golf workout, 244
  running and walking workout, 251
  skiing and skating workout, 247
  tennis workout, 245
"Centers," 6
Chest, 83
  Dégagé, 210, *211*
  Double-Leg Kick, 142, *143*
  Down Dog, 150, *151*
  First and Second Positions, 204–5,
    205, 206, *207*
  Fondu, 212, *213*
  Incline Plank, 192, 193
  90-Degree Front Press Forward,
    214–15, *215*
  Plank with Battements, 148, 149
  Saw, 128, *129*
  Shaving the Head, 224, *224*
  Side Bend, 218, *219*
  Strongman, 216, *216–17*
  Sun Salutation, 194, *194–95*, 196,
    197, 198, *199*
  Tendu en Croix, 208, *209*
Chest Expansion, 220, *221*
Chi, 19
Child's Pose, 144, *145*
Clark, Frank A., 74
Classic Teaser, 180, *181*
  basketball workout, 253
  cycling workout, 249
  golf workout, 244
  running and walking workout, 251
  skiing and skating workout, 247
  tennis workout, 245
Climbing, 256–57
  workout, 257–58
Clothing, workout, 57
Cobra, 138, *139*
  basketball workout, 253
  climbing workout, 257
  cycling workout, 249
  golf workout, 244
  running and walking workout, 251
  skiing and skating workout, 247
  tennis workout, 245
Cohen, Leonard, 75
Coordination

Boomerang, 188, *189*, 190, *191*
Boxing, 222, 223
Chest Expansion, 220, *221*
Dégagé, 210, *211*
Double-Leg Kick, 142, *143*
First and Second Positions, 204–5,
  205, 206, *207*
Fondu, 212, *213*
Head and Body Roll, 96, 97
Hip Flexor Series with Lunges, 200,
  201
90-Degree Front Press Forward,
  214–15, *215*
Open-Leg Rocker, 124, *125*
Open-Leg Rocker Prep, 122, *123*
Pilates benefits, 16
Pillow, 130, *131*
Pull-Down, 94, 95
Seal, 186, *187*
Shaving the Head, 224, *224*
Side Bend, 218, *219*
Single-Leg Pull, 108–9, *109*
Strongman, 216, *216–17*
Swimming, 184, *185*
Tendu en Croix, 208, *209*
"Core muscles," 6, 15
Corkscrew, 126, *127*
  basketball workout, 253
  climbing workout, 257
  cycling workout, 249
  running and walking workout, 251
  skiing and skating workout, 247
  tennis workout, 245
Cramping, foot, 70, 72
Crisscross, 116, *117*
  basketball workout, 253
  climbing workout, 257
  cycling workout, 249
  golf workout, 243
  running and walking workout, 251
  skiing and skating workout, 247
  tennis workout, 245
Cross-training, 15, 241–42
Cycling, 248
  workout, 249–50

Dance, 20–22
  classes, traditional, 21
  Dégagé, 210, 211
  First and Second Positions, 204–5,
    205, 206, *207*

Fondu, 212, *213*
Head and Body Roll, 96, 97
Hip Flexor Series with Lunges, 200,
  201
Pull-Down, 94, 95
Roll-Down, 92–93, *93*
tendu (hard point), *69*, 70, 72–73
Tendu en Croix, 208, *209*
turned out position, 67–68
Dégagé, 210, *211*
  basketball workout, 253
  climbing workout, 257
  cycling workout, 250
  running and walking workout, 251
  skiing and skating workout, 248
  swimming workout, 255
  tennis workout, 246
Dipping Your Foot in the Pool (Pre-
  exercise No. 1), 62
Double-Leg Kick, 142, *143*
  basketball workout, 253
  climbing workout, 257
  cycling workout, 249
  golf workout, 244
  running and walking workout, 251
  skiing and skating workout, 247
  tennis workout, 245
Double-Leg Lower and Lift, 114, *115*
  basketball workout, 253
  climbing workout, 257
  cycling workout, 249
  golf workout, 243
  running and walking workout, 251
  skiing and skating workout, 247
  swimming workout, 255
  tennis workout, 245
Double-Leg Stretch, 110, *111*
  basketball workout, 253
  climbing workout, 257
  cycling workout, 249
  golf workout, 243
  running and walking workout, 251
  skiing and skating workout, 247
  swimming workout, 255
  tennis workout, 245
Down Dog, 150, *151*
  golf workout, 244
  skiing and skating workout, 247
  tennis workout, 245
Down Dog Nose to Knee, 152, *153*
  basketball workout, 253

climbing workout, 257
running and walking workout, 251
swimming workout, 255

Effortless effort, 26, 43–44, 45 (exercise 12)
Einstein, Albert, 75
Energy bath stoppers, 33
Equilibrium, 71. *See also Balance*
Equipment, 58
Establishing the navel-to-spine connection, 26, 41–43 (exercise 11)
   breathing and, 31
Evaluation/placement test, 58–61

Feet
   Cat-Cow Combination, 132, *133*
   cramping, 70, 72
   Dégagé, 210, *211*
   First and Second Positions, 204–5, 205, 206, 207
   flexing the foot, or "look at the heels of your shoes!," 69–70, *69*
   Fondu, 212, *213*
   hard point, or "why should you point your foot like a ballerina when you're never going to wear a tutu?," 69, 70, 72–73
   Incline Plank, 192, 193
   long, loosely pointed foot, 68, *69*
   structural imbalance in body, pain, and alignment of feet, 71
   Tendu en Croix, 208, *209*
Fisher, George, 242
Flat Yoga Press, 146, 147
   basketball workout, 253
   climbing workout, 257
   running and walking workout, 251
   skiing and skating workout, 247
   swimming workout, 255
   tennis workout, 245
Flexibility, 1
   Down Dog Nose to Knee, 152, *153*
   Neck Pull, 154, *155*
   Pilates benefits, 16
   quadriceps-hamstring connection, 80–82
   Rollover, 156, *157*
   Roll-Up, 102, *103*
   Saw, 128, *129*

Scissors, 112, *112*
Fondu, 212, *213*
   basketball workout, 253
   climbing workout, 257
   cycling workout, 250
   running and walking workout, 251
   skiing and skating workout, 248
   swimming workout, 255
   tennis workout, 246

Gentry, Eve, 6–7
Gilbran, Kahlil, xi
Golf, 242–43
   workout, 243–44
"Gospel of Relaxation, The" (James), 27

Habbington, William, 55
Hands, Cat-Cow Combination, 132, *133*
Head and Body Roll, 96, 97
   basketball workout, 253
   climbing workout, 257
   cycling workout, 249
   golf workout, 243
   insight, 96
   running and walking workout, 251
   skiing and skating workout, 247
   swimming workout, 255
   tennis workout, 245
Head Lift, or "Eyes on Your Belly Button" (Pre-exercise No. 2), 62–64
Heart
   breathing exercises and, 34–35
   diaphragm and, 28
   Kapalabhati breathing, 39, 90, *91*
Hip Flexor Series with Lunges, 200, *201*
   basketball workout, 253
   climbing workout, 257
   cycling workout, 249
   running and walking workout, 251
   skiing and skating workout, 248
   swimming workout, 255
Hips
   Bicycle, 168, *169*
   Chest Expansion, 220, *221*
   Crisscross, 116, *117*
   Dégagé, 210, *211*
   Down Dog Nose to Knee, 152, *153*

First and Second Positions, 204–5, 205, 206, 207
Flexor Series with Lunges, 200, *201*
Fondu, 212, *213*
Hot Potato, 174, *175*
Inner Thigh Crossover, 170, *171*
90-Degree Front Press Forward, 214–15, *215*
Pendulum, 164, *165*
Pilates benefits, 16
Ronde de Jambe, 172, *173*
Shaving the Head, 224, *224*
Side Bend, 218, *219*
Single-Leg Pull, 108–9, *109*
Strongman, 216, *216–17*
Sun Salutation, 194, *194–95*, 196, 197, 198, *199*
Tendu en Croix, 208, *209*
Toss-Up, 166, *167*
Hot Potato, 174, *175*
Hug, 226, *227*
Hundred, 98, 99
   basketball workout, 253
   climbing workout, 257
   cycling workout, 249
   golf workout, 243
   insight, 99
   preparation: Campfire Breathing, or seated preparation for the Hundred Breath (Pre-exercise No. 6), 73–74
   preparation: Head Lift, or "Eyes on Your Belly Button" (Pre-exercise No. 2), 62–64
   running and walking workout, 251
   skiing and skating workout, 247
   swimming workout, 255
   tennis workout, 245

Incline Plank, 192, 193
   climbing workout, 257
   swimming workout, 255
   tennis workout, 245
Inner Thigh Crossover, 170, *171*
   golf workout, 244
Insights, 74–82
   Active Cat with Yoga Press, 136, *137*
   Active Moving Cat, 134
   Alternate Nostril Breathing, 232
   Arm Circles, 228

Bicycle, 168
Boomerang, 190
Boxing, 222
Cat-Cow Combination, 132
Chest Expansion, 220
Child's Pose, 144
Classic Teaser, 180
Cobra, 138
Corkscrew, 126
Crisscross, 116
Dégagé, 210
Double-Leg Kick, 142
Double-Leg Lower and Lift, 114
Double-Leg Stretch, 110
Down Dog, 150
Down Dog Nose to Knee, 152
First and Second Positions, 206
Flat Yoga Press, 147
Fondu, 212
Head and Body Roll, 96
Hot Potato, 174
Hug, 226
The Hundred, 99
Inner Thigh Crossover, 170
Jackknife, 176
Kapalabhati breathing, 90
Leg Circles, 105
meditation, 235
muscle pairings, 78–82, 83, 84
Neck Pull, 154, 155
90-Degree Front Press Forward, 215
Pelvic Lift with Leg Extension, 118
Pendulum, 164
Pillow, 130, 131
Plank with Battements, 148
post-sculpting relaxation, 231
Pre-Roll-Up, 100
Pull-Down, 94
Roll-Down, 93
Rolling like a Ball, 107
Rollover, 156
Roll-Up, 102
Ronde de Jambe, 172
Savasana, 236
Saw, 128
Scissors, 112
Seal, 186, 187
Seated Forward Bend, 160, 161
Shaving the Head, 224
Side Bend, 218
Single-Bent-Leg Teaser, 178

Single-Leg Kick, 140
Single-Leg Pull, 109
spinal articulation, 74–78
Spine Stretch Forward, 121
Spine Twist, 158
Strongman, 217
Sun Salutation, 198
Sun Salutation Warrior II, 202
Swimming, 184
Tendu en Croix, 208
Toss-Up, 166
Intuitive integration, 26, 48–49
quality and quantity with intuitive
integration, 49–50 (exercise 14)

Jackknife, 176, 177
climbing workout, 257
swimming workout, 255
James, William, 17, 27, 43, 89, 239,
269
Joints, Pilates benefits, 16
Jong, K. T., 53

Kapalabhati breathing, breath of fire,
19, 30
basketball workout, 253
climbing workout, 257
cycling workout, 249
exercise 9, 39, 90, 91
golf workout, 243
insight, 90
running and walking workout, 251
skiing and skating workout, 247
swimming workout, 255 tennis workout, 245
Kries, Jennifer
ballet instruction, 5
childhood, 5
"Conditioning Class," New York City
Ballet's Summer Intensive, 5–7
contact information, 271
healing and, 8
hip injury, 7, 8
Method created by, 10
Pilates certification and study by,
9–10
Pilates, discovery of, 5–7
as Pilates instructor, 8, 9–10
teachers studied with, 6, 9

yoga and mind-body integration,
17–18, 20
yoga training of, 7–8

Leg Circles, 104–5, 105
cycling workout, 249
Legs (abductor, adductors, hamstrings,
quadriceps, rotator muscles), 83,
84
Active Moving Cat, 134, 135
Bicycle, 168, 169
Boomerang, 188, 189, 190, 191
Boxing, 222, 223
Cobra, 138, 139
Corkscrew, 126, 127
Crisscross, 116, 117
Dégagé, 210, 211
Double-Leg Kick, 142, 143
Down Dog, 150, 151
Down Dog Nose to Knee, 152, 153
First and Second Positions, 204–5,
205, 206, 207
Flat Yoga Press, 146, 147
Fondu, 212, 213
Head and Body Roll, 96, 97
Hip Flexor Series with Lunges, 200,
201
Hot Potato, 174, 175
Incline Plank, 192, 193
Inner Thigh Crossover, 170, 171
Leg Circles, 104–5, 105
long, loosely pointed foot, 68
Neck Pull, 154, 155
90-Degree Front Press Forward,
214–15, 215
Open-Leg Rocker, 124, 125
Open-Leg Rocker Prep, 122, 123
Pelvic Lift with Leg Extension, 118,
119
Pendulum, 164, 165
Pilates benefits, 16
Plank with Battements, 148, 149
Pull-Down, 94, 95
quadriceps-hamstring connection,
80–82
Roll-Down, 92, 93
Rollover, 156, 157
Roll-Up, 102, 103
Ronde de Jambe, 172, 173
Saw, 128, 129

Scissors, 112, *112*
Seated Forward Bend, 160, *161*
Side Bend, 218, *219*
Single-Leg Kick, 140, *141*
Single-Leg Pull, 108–9, *109*
Spine Stretch Forward, 120, *121*
Spine Twist, 158, *159*
Strongman, 216, *216–17*
Sun Salutation, 194, *194–95*, 196,
    197, 198, *199*
Sun Salutation Warrior II, 202, *203*
Swimming, 184, *185*
Tendu en Croix, 208, *209*
Toss-Up, 166, *167*
turned out position and, 67
"Lengthening through," 68
Level 1 exercises, 59, 60
    Active Moving Cat, 134, *135*
    Alternate Nostril Breathing, 232–33,
        232–33
    Cat-Cow Combination, 132, *133*
    Child's Pose, 144, *145*
    Cobra, 138, *139*
    Dipping Your Foot in the Pool (Pre-
        exercise No. 1), 62
    Down Dog, 150, *151*
    First Position, 204–5, *205*
    Flat Yoga Press, 146, 147
    Head and Body Roll, 96, 97
    Head Lift, or "Eyes on Your Belly
        Button" (Pre-exercise No. 2),
        62–64
    Hundred, 98–99, 99
    Kapalabhati Breathing, 90, *91*
    Leg Circles, 104–5, *105*
    Meditation, 234, *235*
    90-Degree Front Press Forward,
        214, *215*
    Open-Leg Rocker Prep, 122, *123*
    Pendulum, 164, *165*
    Pillow, 130, *131*
    Pre-Roll-Up, 100, *101*
    Pull-Down, 94, 95
    Roll-Down, 92, 93
    Rolling like a Ball, 106–7, *107*
    Roll-Up, 102, *103*
    Savasana, 236, *237*
    Seal, 186, *187*
    Seated Forward Bend, 160, *161*
    Second Position, 206, *207*
    Single-Bent-Leg Teaser, 178, *179*

Single-Leg Kick, 140, *141*
Single-Leg Pull, 108–9, *109*
Spine Stretch Forward, 120, *121*
Strongman, 216, *216–17*
Sun Salutation, 194, *194–95*, 196,
    197, 198, *199*
Sun Salutation Warrior II, 202, *203*
Swimming, 184, *185*
Tendu en Croix, 208, *209*
Toss-Up, 166, *167*
Level 2, 60
    Active Cat with Yoga Press, 136, *137*
    Arms-to-Ears Teaser, 182, *183*
    Bicycle, 168, *169*
    Boxing, 222
    Chest Expansion, 220, *221*
    Classic Teaser, 180, *181*
    Corkscrew, 126, *127*
    Crisscross, 116, *117*
    Dégagé, 210, *211*
    Double-Leg Kick, 142, *143*
    Double-Leg Lower and Lift, 114,
        115
    Double-Leg Stretch, 110, *111*
    Down Dog Nose to Knee, 152, *153*
    Fondu, 212, *213*
    Hip Flexor Series with Lunges, 200,
        201
    Inner Thigh Crossover, 170, *171*
    Neck Pull, 154, *155*
    Pelvic Lift with Leg Extension, 118,
        119
    Plank with Battements, 148, *149*
    Saw, 128, *129*
    Scissors, 112, *112*
    Shaving the Head, 224, *224*
    Side Bend, 218, *219*
    Spine Twist, 158, *159*
Level 3, 60
    Arm Circles, 228, *229*
    Boomerang, 188, *189*, 190, *191*
    Hot Potato, 174, *175*
    Hug, 226, 227
    Incline Plank, 192, 193
    Jackknife, 176, *177*
    Rollover, 156, *157*
    Ronde de Jambe, 172, *173*
Levels
    assessment form, 271–73
    evaluation/placement test, 58–59
    general information, 87

progressing to higher, 87–88
    time spent at each level, 59–61
Location of workout, 57
Lung capacity
    The Hundred, 98–99, *99*
    Kapalabhati breathing, 39, 90, *91*

Magic triangle, 13
Mandela, Nelson, 85, 263
Meditation, 26, 53–54, 54 (exercise
    17), 234, 235
    alternate nostril breathing and, 40
        (exercise 10), 232–33, *232–33*
    basketball workout, 253
    climbing workout, 257
    cycling workout, 250
    golf workout, 244
    running and walking workout, 251
    skiing and skating workout, 248
    swimming workout, 255
    tennis workout, 246
Method Workout
    abdominal strength stressed, 1
    assessment form, 271–73
    background of and benefits, 1–2, 10
    balance and moderation in, 44
    benefits, 266–68
    body transformation with, 266
    breathing, 27–40, 32
    complete listing of all exercises,
        88–89
    dance in, 20–22
    effortless effort (command without
        tension), 43–45
    equipment needed, 58
    establishing the navel-to-spine con-
        nection, 41–43
    flexibility and, 1
    insights, 74–82
    intuitive integration, 48–49
    level, determining (evaluation/place-
        ment test), 58–61
    level, progressing to higher, 87–88
    meditation, 53–54, 54 (exercise 17),
        234, 235
    mind-body approach of, 10, 20
    nine essential elements, 25–54
    as philosophy, 1, 42, 76–77, 265
    Pilates in, 16–17
    posture improvement, 76
    pre-exercises, 61–74, 87

principle of opposition, 45, *46*, 47
  (exercise 13), 65, 82
quality and quantity with intuitive
  integration, 49–50 (exercise 14)
quality versus quantity, 48
routines, creating your own, 87
speed of results, 58
sports performance boosted by,
  241–42
sports workouts, 242–58
strength and endurance, 1
tempo and dynamic, 51–53 (exercise
  16)
time-saving workouts, 258–61
transitions, 50–51 (exercise 15)
what to wear, 57
when to workout, 57–58
where to workout, 57
yoga in, 17–20
See also Breathing; Effortless effort;
  Establishing the navel-to-spine
  connection; Insights; Intuitive
  integration; Pre-exercises;
  Principle of opposition; Quality
  versus quantity; Tempo and
  dynamic; Transitions; *specific
  exercises*
Mind-body integration, 7, 8, 17–18, 20
  breath as bridge, 27
  posture, effect of negative experi-
    ences and feelings on spine,
    76–77
  spinal articulation, as self-care,
    77–78
Moore, George, 1
Mountain Pose, 66–67
Mula bhanda (anal lock; exercise 3),
  34–35
Muscles, *83, 84*
  cramping, 70, 72
  creating bulk, concerns about, 82
  fatiguing, 82
  latissimus-trapezius connection,
    78–80
  quadriceps-hamstring connection,
    80–82
Music, 94

Neck, *83, 84*
  Cat-Cow Combination, 132, *133*
  Chest Expansion, 220, *221*

Child's Pose, 144, *145*
  Head and Body Roll, 96, *97*
  Neck Pull, 154, *155*
  Roll-Down, 92, *93*
  Rolling like a Ball, 106–7, *107*
  Spine Stretch Forward, 120, *121*
Neck Pull, 154, *155*
  basketball workout, 253
  climbing workout, 257
  running and walking workout, 251
  skiing and skating workout, 247
  swimming workout, 255
New York City Ballet, 5
90-Degree Front Press Forward,
  214–15, *215*

On the Fly (time-saving workouts)
  Workout I (beginner), 258–59
  Workout II (intermediate and
    advanced), 260–61
Open-Leg Rocker, 124, *125*
  basketball workout, 253
  climbing workout, 257
  running and walking workout, 251
  skiing and skating workout, 247
  swimming workout, 255
Open-Leg Rocker Prep, 122, *123*

Pain
  lack of equilibrium and feet, 71
  spinal articulation (posture) and,
    74–78
  Swimming exercise, 184, *185*
  Pelvic Lift with Leg Extension, 118,
    119
  basketball workout, 253
  climbing workout, 257
  cycling workout, 249
  running and walking workout, 251
  skiing and skating workout, 247
  swimming workout, 255
  tennis workout, 245
Pendulum, 164, *165*
  golf workout, 244
Pennsylvania Ballet, 5
Pilates, Joseph, 14–15
  Balanchine and, 6
  Gentry, Eve, and, 6
  quotes from, 14
  wife, Clara, 14
Pilates method

Arm Circles, 228, *229*
Arms-to-Ears Teaser, 182, *183*
as "Art of Contrology," 7
athletes, use of for cross-training,
  15, 241–42
benefits, 7, 16
Boomerang, 188, *189*, 190, *191*
Boxing, 222, *223*
Chest Expansion, 220, *221*
Classic Teaser, 180, *181*
Corkscrew, 126, *127*
Crisscross, 116, *117*
Double-Leg Kick, 142, *143*
Double-Leg Lower and Lift, 114,
  115
Double-Leg Stretch, 110, *111*
Hug, 226, *227*
The Hundred, 6, 63–64, 73–74,
  98–99, *99*
incremental nature of, 15–16
injury prevention with, 15
Jackknife, 176, *177*
Leg Circles, 104–5, *105*
mat work, 16
Neck Pull, 154, *155*
90-Degree Front Press Forward,
  214–15, *215*
Open-Leg Rocker, 124, *125*
Open-Leg Rocker Prep, 122, *123*
Pelvic Lift with Leg Extension, 118,
  119
Pillow, 130, *131*
Plank with Battements, 148, *149*
Pre-Roll-Up, 100, *101*
Rolling like a Ball, 106–7, *107*
Rollover, 156, *157*
Roll-Up, 102, *103*
Saw, 128, *129*
Scissors, 112, *112*
Seal, 186, *187*
Shaving the Head, 224, *224*
Side Bend, 218, *219*
Single-Bent-Leg Teaser, 178, *179*
Single-Leg Kick, 140, *141*
Single-Leg Pull, 108–9, *109*
Spine Stretch Forward, 120, *121*
Spine Twist, 158, *159*
Swimming, 184, *185*
tripod stance, 66
Pillow, 130, *131*
  golf workout, 244

Pineapple Dance Center, 7
Plank with Battements, 148, *149*
  basketball workout, 253
  climbing workout, 257
  cycling workout, 249
  running and walking workout, 251
  skiing and skating workout, 247
  swimming workout, 255
  tennis workout, 245
Plié series
  basketball workout, 253
  climbing workout, 257
  cycling workout, 250
  Dégagé, 210, *211*
  First and Second Positions, 204–5,
    205, 206, 207
  Fondu, 212, *213*
  golf workout, 244
  running and walking workout, 251
  skiing and skating workout, 248
  swimming workout, 255
  Tendu en Croix, 208, *209*
  tennis workout, 245
Poe, Edgar Allan, 256
Point of Control (Pre-exercise No. 1),
  64–65
Point, Flex, and Lengthen (Pre-exercise No. 5), 68–70, *69*, 72–73
  cramping, 70, 72
  flexing the foot, or "look at the heels
    of your shoes!," 69–70, *69*
  hard point, or "why should you point
    your foot like a ballerina when
    you're never going to wear a
    tutu?," *69*, 70, 72–73
  long, loosely pointed foot, 68, *69*
Posture
  Bicycle, 168, *169*
  Cat-Cow Combination, 132, *133*
  Cobra, 138, *139*
  Flat Yoga Press, 146, 147
  Method Workout, improvement of
    and, 76
  90-Degree Front Press Forward,
    214–15, *215*
  Pendulum, 164, *165*
  Pilates benefits, 16
  Shaving the Head, 224, *224*
  Side Bend, 218, *219*
  spinal articulation, 74–78
  Spine Stretch Forward, 120, *121*

Toss-Up, 166, *167*
"Powerhouse," 6, 15
Pranayama, 27
Pre-exercises, 87
  benefits, 61
  No. 1: Dipping Your Foot in the Pool,
    62
  No. 2: Head Lift, or "Eyes on Your
    Belly Button," 62–64
  No. 3: Point of Control, 64–65
  No. 4: Standing Positions, 65–68
  No. 5: Point, Flex, and Lengthen,
    68–70, *69*, 72–73
  No. 6: Campfire Breathing, 73–74
Preparation for working out
  clothing, 57
  equipment, 58
  frequency, 57
  location, 57
  pre-exercises, 61–74, 87
  time of day, 58
Pre-Roll-Up, 100, *101*
  basketball workout, 253
  climbing workout, 257
  cycling workout, 249
  evaluation/placement test, 58–61
  golf workout, 243
  insight, 100
  running and walking workout, 251
  skiing and skating workout, 247
  swimming workout, 255
  tennis workout, 245
Principle of opposition, 26, 45, *46*, 65,
  82
  exercise for, *46, 47*
Prophet, The (Gibran), xi
Proust, Marcel, 11
Pull-Down, 94, *95*
  basketball workout, 253
  climbing workout, 257
  cycling workout, 249
  insight, 94
  running and walking workout, 251
  skiing and skating workout, 247
  swimming workout, 255
  tennis workout, 245

Qi gong, 27
Quality versus quantity, 26, 48
  with intuitive integration, 49–50 (exer-
    cise 14)

Range of motion, 7
Roll-Down, 92, *93*
  basketball workout, 253
  cycling workout, 249
  insight, 93
  running and walking workout, 251
  skiing and skating workout, 247
  swimming workout, 255
Rolling like a Ball, 106, *107*
  basketball workout, 253
  climbing workout, 257
  cycling workout, 249
  golf workout, 243
  insight, 107
  running and walking workout, 251
  skiing and skating workout, 247
  swimming workout, 255
  tennis workout, 245
Rollover, 156, *157*
  basketball workout, 253
  climbing workout, 257
  cycling workout, 249
  running and walking workout, 251
  skiing and skating workout, 247
  swimming workout, 255
Roll-Up, 102, *103*
  basketball workout, 253
  climbing workout, 257
  cycling workout, 249
  golf workout, 243
  insight, 102
  running and walking workout, 251
  skiing and skating workout, 247
  swimming workout, 255
  tennis workout, 245
Running and walking, 250–51
  workout, 251–52

Savasana, 236, *237*
  basketball workout, 253
  climbing workout, 257
  cycling workout, 249
  golf workout, 244
  running and walking workout, 251
  skiing and skating workout, 248
  tennis workout, 246
  swimming workout, 255
Saw, 128, *129*
  basketball workout, 253
  climbing workout, 257
  golf workout, 244

running and walking workout, 251
skiing and skating workout, 247
swimming workout, 255
tennis workout, 245
School of American Ballet, 5
Scissors, 112, *112*
  basketball workout, 253
  climbing workout, 257
  cycling workout, 249
  golf workout, 243
  running and walking workout, 251
  skiing and skating workout, 247
  swimming workout, 255
  tennis workout, 245
Sculpting body, Pilates benefits, 16.
    See also Standing sculpting series
Seal, 186, *187*
  golf workout, 244
  tennis workout, 245
Seated Forward Bend, 160, *161*
  basketball workout, 253
  climbing workout, 257
  cycling workout, 249
  running and walking workout, 251
  skiing and skating workout, 247
  swimming workout, 255
Shaving the Head, 224, *224*
Shaw, George Bernard, 3
Shoulders (trapezius muscles), 83, 84
  Boxing, 222, 223
  Cat-Cow Combination, 132, *133*
  Chest Expansion, 220, *221*
  Child's Pose, 144, *145*
  Dégagé, 210, *211*
  Double-Leg Kick, 142, *143*
  Down Dog, 150, 151
  First and Second Positions, 204–5,
    205, 206, 207
  Fondu, 212, *213*
  golf workout, 244
  Head and Body Roll, 96, 97
  Hug, 226, 227
  The Hundred, 98, 99
  Incline Plank, 192, 193
  latissimus-trapezius connection,
    78–80
  90-Degree Front Press Forward,
    214–15, *215*
  Plank with Battements, 148, *149*
  Roll-Down, 92, *93*
  Saw, 128, *129*

Shaving the Head, 224, *224*
Side Bend, 218, *219*
Spine Stretch Forward, 120, *121*
Spine Twist, 158, *159*
Sun Salutation, 194, *194–95*, 196,
    197, 198, *199*
Side Bend, 218, *219*
Side Series, 162
  basketball workout, 253
  climbing workout, 257
  cycling workout, 249
  golf workout, 244
  helpful hints, 162–63
  Hot Potato, 174, *175*
  Inner Thigh Crossover, 170, *171*
  Jackknife, 176, *177*
  Pendulum, 164, *165*
  Ronde de Jambe, 172, *173*
  running and walking workout, 251
  skiing and skating workout, 247
  swimming workout, 255
  tennis workout, 245
  Toss-Up, 166, *167*
Single-Bent-Leg Teaser, 178, *179*
  basketball workout, 253
  cycling workout, 249
  golf workout, 244
  running and walking workout, 251
  skiing and skating workout, 247
  tennis workout, 245
Single-Leg Kick, 140, *141*
  basketball workout, 253
  climbing workout, 257
  cycling workout, 249
  running and walking workout, 251
  skiing and skating workout, 247
  swimming workout, 255
  tennis workout, 245
Single-Leg Pull, 108–9, *109*
  basketball workout, 253
  climbing workout, 257
  cycling workout, 249
  golf workout, 243
  skiing and skating workout, 247
  swimming workout, 255
  tennis workout, 245
Skiing and Skating, 246–46
  workout, 247–48
Spine and spinal articulation, 74–78
  benefits, 75–76
  Cat-Cow Combination, 132, *133*

Child's Pose, 144, *145*
Jackknife, 176, *177*
Pre-Roll-Up, 100, *101*
Roll-Down, 92, *93*
Rolling like a Ball, 106–7, *107*
"rolling through," 75
Roll-Up, 102, *103*
Seated Forward Bend, 160, *161*
Spine Stretch Forward, 120, *121*
  basketball workout, 253
  climbing workout, 257
  cycling workout, 249
  golf workout, 243
  running and walking workout, 251
  skiing and skating workout, 247
  swimming workout, 255
  tennis workout, 245
Spine Twist, 158, *159*
  basketball workout, 253
  climbing workout, 257
  cycling workout, 249
  golf workout, 244
  running and walking workout, 251
  skiing and skating workout, 247
  swimming workout, 255
  tennis workout, 245
Stamina, 7
  dance and, 20
Standing Positions (Pre-exercise No.4),
    65–68
  parallel, 66–67
  tripod, 66
  turned out, 67–68
Standing sculpting series, 214–231
  Arm Circles, 228, 229
  basketball workout, 253
  Boxing, 222, 223
  Chest Expansion, 220, *221*
  climbing workout, 257
  cycling workout, 249
  golf workout, 244
  Hug, 226, 227
  90-Degree Front Press Forward,
    214–15, *215*
  post-sculpting relaxation, 230
  Shaving the Head, 224, *224*
  running and walking workout, 251
  skiing and skating workout, 248
  Side Bend, 218, *219*
  Strongman, 216, *216–17*
  swimming workout, 255

tennis workout, 246
Strength, Pilates benefits, 16
Strongman, 216, *216–17*
Sun Salutation, 19, 194, *194–95*, 196, *197*, 198, *199*
  basketball workout, 253
  climbing workout, 257
  cycling workout, 249
  running and walking workout, 251
  skiing and skating workout, 247
  swimming workout, 255
  tennis workout, 246
  Warrior II, 202, *203*
Sun Ssu-mo, 23
Swimming, 184, *185*
  basketball workout, 253
  climbing workout, 257
  cycling workout, 249
  golf workout, 244
  running and walking workout, 251
  skiing and skating workout, 247
  swimming workout, 255
  tennis workout, 245
Swimming (sport of), 254–55
  workout, 255–56
Symmetry, 69, 82
  Pelvic Lift with Leg Extension, 118, *119*

Tao, 23
Teaser series
  Arms-to-Ears Teaser, 182, *183*
  Classic Teaser, 180, *181*
  cycling workout, 249
  golf workout, 244
  Single-Bent-Leg Teaser, 178, *179*
  skiing and skating workout, 247

swimming workout, 255
  tennis workout, 245
Tempo and dynamic, 26, 51–53 (exercise 16)
Tendu (hard point), *69*, 70, 72–73
Tendu en Croix, 208, *209*
  basketball workout, 253
  climbing workout, 257
  cycling workout, 250
  golf workout, 244
  running and walking workout, 251
  skiing and skating workout, 248
  swimming workout, 255
  tennis workout, 245
Tennis, 244–45
  workout, 245–46
Throat lock (exercise 5), 35–36
Toss-Up, 166, *167*
Transitions, 26, 50–51 (exercise 15)

Ujjayi breathing, 19, 30, 38 (exercise 8)
Upper body
  Arm Circles, 228, 229
  Boxing, 222, *223*
  Chest Expansion, 220, *221*
  Down Dog Nose to Knee, 152, *153*
  Flat Yoga Press, 146, 147
  Incline Plank, 192, 193
  Plank with Battements, 148, *149*
  sculpting series, 13
  strength, 8, 13
  Sun Salutation Warrior II, 202, *203*
  yoga asanas (postures) and, 19–20

Van Dyke, Henry, 271
Vonnegut, Kurt, 254

Waist (infraspinatus, serratus anterior, teres major), 15, 83, *84*
Walk (gait pattern), 76

Yoga, 17–20
  Active Cat with Yoga Press, 136, *137*
  Active Moving Cat, 134, *135*
  alternate nostril breathing, 40 (exercise 10), 232–33, *232–33*
  asanas, 19
  ashtanga, 18
  body-mind approach of, 17, 20
  breathing, 7, 18–19, 29–40
  Cat-Cow Combination, 132, *133*
  Child's Pose, 144, *145*
  Cobra, 138, *139*
  Down Dog, 150, *151*
  Down Dog Nose to Knee, 152, *153*
  Flat Yoga Press, 146, 147
  hatha, 18
  Hip Flexor Series with Lunges, 200, 201
  Incline Plank, 192, 193
  Iyengar, 18
  meditation, 234–35, *235*
  mula bhanda (exercise 3), 34–35
  parallel stance (Mountain Pose), 66–67
  Pelvic Lift with Leg Extension, 118, *119*
  Roll-Down, 92–93, *93*
  Savasana, 236, *237*
  Seated Forward Bend, 160, *161*
  Sun Salutation, 19, 194, *194–95*, 196, *197*, 198, *199*
  Sun Salutation Warrior II, 202, *203*
  upper body strength and, 19–20

ABOUT THE AUTHOR

JENNIFER KRIES, native New Yorker, dancer, choreographer, Master Instructor, orator and fitness celebrity made her professional debut at sixteen in Balanchine's *Serenade* with Edward Villella's Eglevsky Ballet. She trained with The School of American Ballet and is a former member of the Pennsylvania Ballet and Philadelphia's Waves Jazz Dance Company. Her choreography and teaching credits include John Leguizamo's FOX show "House of Buggin," New York City Ballet, Hubbard Street Chicago and Pennsylvania Ballet Summer residencies, and Bat Sheva Dance Company, Tel Aviv. Kries studied with three of Joseph Pilates' original disciples, Eve Gentry, Romana Kryzanowska, and Ron Fletcher. The synergy of her pilates and dance background, coupled with her intensive study of anatomy and Yoga (including Hatha, Iyengar, Kundalini, and Ashtanga), led to the creation of *Jennifer Kries' Pilates Plus Method.*

Jennifer is the artistic director and founder of Contemporary Dance Theatre New York and the Founder of the Balanced Body Center at New York's World Gym where she educates both teachers and the public in her Pilates Plus Method for rehabilitation and strength training. Her mat class was voted one of America's Top Ten Group Classes by Shape Magazine and has since been introduced to a wide range of public and private fitness facilities across the United States and the world.

Jennifer Kries is featured in seven popular, award-winning fitness videos in the series, The Method. She received Fitness Magazine's "Best Mind-Body Video Award" in 1999. She created, choreographed and starred in fifty two episodes of FOX/ Fit TV's Alternative Health and Fitness Series, The Method Show, which aired nationwide. A new series of three videos, *Jennifer Kries' Pilates Method*, was just released and is available in stores and through www.CollageVideo.com.